I Wish I Were A Leper

The Diary of One Couple's Struggle
with Fear, Faith and Alzheimer's

VINCE O'ROURKE

I Wish I Were a Leper: The Diary of One Couple's
Struggle with Fear, Faith and Alzheimer's
Vince O'Rourke © 2024

All rights reserved. No part of this book may be used or reproduced by any means, graphic, electronic, or mechanical, including photocopying, recording, taping or by any information storage retrieval system without the written permission of the author except in the case of brief quotations embodied in critical articles and reviews.

Because of the dynamic nature of the Internet, any web addresses or links contained in this book may have changed since publication and may no longer be valid. The views expressed in this work are solely those of the author and do not necessarily reflect the views of the publisher, and the publisher hereby disclaims any responsibility for them.

Printed in the United States of America

To Contact the author go to: vlorourke@bigpond.com or
carersoutlook@gmail.com

Library of Congress Control Number:	2024935338
Paperback:	978-1-952648-89-2
Hardcover:	978-1-952648-88-5

Contents

Preface	ix
Introduction	xiii
Chapter 1 The Journey Begins	1
Chapter 2 1999 Testing and Hoping	7
Chapter 3 2000 Towards Fulltime Caring	21
Chapter 4 2001 Towards Total Reliance	35
Chapter 5 2002 An Adult as Child	55
Chapter 6 2003 Securing Regular Assistance	81
Chapter 7 2004 A Hard Day's Night	115
Chapter 8 2005 Final Months at Home	143
Chapter 9 The Nandeebie Period	169
Chapter 10 Epilogue Farewell Margaret	205
Postscript	215
Glossary	219
Relevant Contacts	221

Preface

When my dear wife Margaret eventually died, at age 67, from the inevitable consequences of Alzheimer's disease, I was devastated. I had nursed her in our home for many years and finally had to place her in the care of others in a nursing home of our choice. My grief and anger were so great I felt I had to find some way of coping.

This book began as my own personal way of dealing with the nine years of watching the most precious gift in my life being ever so gradually taken from me. I felt I needed to relive our journey and be open to the messages it contained. It gave me a reason to wake up each day amongst other things.

My effort to write was greatly aided by the daily diaries I had kept throughout the journey. I could never have done it without them. When there is a lot of pain in one's journey, memory seems to gain in its selectivity. There was indeed so very much that I had forgotten. I decided early on to write as truthful an account as I could; aided by my diary entries. That meant that I was forced to reread the diaries and re-experience the pain and the loss again.

Strangely, through the pain of revisiting our journey, I grew to appreciate the struggle that we had experienced and felt a little more at peace with my efforts to care for my Margaret in keeping with the vows freely undertaken when we were first married in 1965. At the time of writing I had no intention of sharing our journey with anyone other than eventually my three daughters.

One of the positive outcomes of this period of my life was reconnecting with my sisters. When they heard of my writing they prevailed upon me to read it to them. I finally agreed to do so over a period of months. It was a way for me to do a first edit. They were very impressed with what I had written and found they had little knowledge of all that the journey had meant for both Margaret and me.

When I had the story in its completed form, I gave a copy to each of my three daughters to read. It was an eye opener for them too. They now joined with my sisters in asking that I consider how our journey could be of assistance to many others who would find themselves in the carer's role. I had many reservations about so revealing to a wider public what our journey with early onset Alzheimer's entailed.

I now asked two friends who helped care for Margaret in her last twelve to fifteen months in the nursing home to read the book for me from a professional standpoint. Their encouragement to publish for a wider audience beyond family and friends was instrumental in my getting to this point.

My hope is that this account of our personal journey with Alzheimer's will be a help for all carers, whether non professional like myself or professionals, as are those who work in the nursing care industry. I would wish for a politician or two to read it and to come to a clearer understanding of what the life of the carer entails, to see the real need for an ever increasing supply of nursing homes and in-home support. Further I would hope that people who read this book may come to an understanding of the nature of this terrible disease and the need that both sufferer and carer have for support and acceptance.

As with many books, this book has a number of themes. I grew aware in the reliving of our journey how important a place faith and prayer had played. God is an easy target when one is hurt and angry. Underlying the more obvious story is my particular struggle with my God in times of grief and suffering. Some readers may find comfort in the very humanness of my confrontations with my God. I hope that the reader will come to appreciate that this account of our long farewell is also one of the unconditional love two people can share in marriage.

I would want to thank a number of people who have helped me get to this point. Our wonderful daughters Maree, Megan and Anne have always been my tower of strength. Their ongoing support would have been far more limited but for the understanding of their husbands - Michael, Ben and Richard. Thanks to my sisters, Colleen Angwin and Helen Tracey, who were so patient in listening to me read the first of many drafts. Thanks also to Catherine Shirlock and Annette McAlpine whose encouragement, from a professional care giver's point of view, was instrumental in my publishing.

Two other people have read the manuscript for me and then encouraged me to publish. Professor Frank Pignatelli from Scotland, a long time friend and colleague, knew Margaret long before she contracted this disease. Fr John Chalmers is a person with whom I have had contact over many years and for whom Margaret and I helped produce a series of talks for the preparation of engaged couples some thirty years ago.

Finally I wish to record my thanks to Maurice Ryan who helped me through the maze which is the lot of the neophyte in the world of publishing.

Vince O'Rourke
January 2008

Introduction

Many years ago I read Stephen Covey's "The Seven Habits of Highly Effective People". I thought he presented a number of wonderful insights into the human dimension of life. Among a number of things, I found myself drawn to what he set out as our four basic needs viz., to live, to love, to learn and to leave a legacy.

When my beautiful wife died in October 2006 I applied these four aspects of human need to Margaret's life. They sat neatly with various aspects of her journey on this earth. In my thinking I came to better understand that meeting such needs is not accomplished alone. We live a life of relationships and through these, or in spite of them at times, we advance through life.

Our relationship through 41 years of marriage was a very special gift. It was a gift which prepared us to journey together through the 10 years when Margaret was beset by early onset Alzheimer's disease. That journey affected many people in ways we would never have guessed. In the light of that I was moved to write of our journey with Alzheimer's.

I am a diary or journal writer. For 20 years I have written about aspects of my daily life. It has become an integral part of each day. I have therefore recorded a great deal about the years Margaret and I spent trying to cope with all that a disease like Alzheimer's brings for both sufferer and carer. My diaries form the basis for this book.

As I read through my diaries to write our story, I saw connections in events that had eluded me during the course of our journey. The retracing of our steps together has helped me face the depth of loss that followed upon Margaret's death. It has also reawakened in me the realization that throughout our lives we have tried to assist in the education and development of others. I saw that to set down the joys and the pains of our experience would add to Margaret's already outstanding legacy.

I cared for Margaret in our own home for 7.5 years until July 2005. When she entered a nursing home my role as carer changed; it did not end. I was with her every day for 3 – 4 hours until her death on 10 October 2006. The caring role is difficult and I am sure the experience of each carer is rather unique. Nevertheless, I hope that my part in our story may be of assistance to all carers and particularly to men in that role.

It was difficult to determine to write of our journey. It is by its nature very personal and private. I would never wish to do anything that may lessen the respect held for my Margaret or our family. However to tell of our journey I have been totally honest, at least as I experienced it. It is not a journey to be envied. It is a journey of love, loss and service made by two very human people.

I have not tried to write a clinical account of the progress of a disease. That would not fall within my competence. This is simply a real life account told through the notations made daily in my diaries. I have not amended any aspect of the diary notations. What I wrote is what I wrote.

My hope is that, through the recording of our journey with Alzheimer's, other carers may find that they are not alone in their journey, that help is at hand, that knowledge about the progression of the disease may help in facing and planning for each new challenge, that deep and abiding love will give them the strength to cope with whatever life throws at them. I also hope it may give insights to others such as doctors, nurses and nursing home staff as well as friends and relatives of those who suffer or are carers.

Alzheimer's is a disease on the increase. The more we can appreciate its progression and effects the better we may deal with it in the years ahead.

Chapter 1

The Journey Begins

At precisely 1.15pm on Tuesday October 10, 2006 my beautiful wife of 41 years, Margaret Mary O'Rourke, completed her final struggle against Alzheimer's disease and its complications. Pneumonia, often the direct cause of death in such cases, had its day. As she breathed her last, surrounded by her family, there was no blast of trumpets, no harps or angels, but those present felt a clear sense of her spirit, of her true self, departing gently from her shell of a body. It was her belief and my own that she would go to a place of peace and love. She would forever rest in God's gentle presence.

Margaret's dying was the inevitable conclusion of a process which had begun at least eight years earlier when she was 59. It was not an ending that had ever crossed our minds in the years leading up to that. In all truth I was sure that it would be my lot to die first. Selfishly I thought Margaret's gentleness would befit her in a role of nurse for me. I had not counted on God's sense of humour. I got through my heart attack in 1996 and was blest with good health thereafter because I, the short fused and impatient one in our relationship, was to be called to do the nursing, the caring.

I have absolutely no doubt that the act of caring has to be premised on love. What caring calls one to goes beyond any norms of everyday human behaviour. One can fail often enough even when love for the one needing care is unconditional. The reward is in believing that you are doing your best to express your love. I was called to guard my loved one's dignity as a human being, while watching a disease gradually strip her of the very functions of life we take for granted.

How and why two particular people grow to love one another is, for me, one of the mysteries of life. I choose to believe that the hand of God can be seen in our story.

Margaret was the eldest of seven children whose mother was a long-time friend of my mother. My mother had been bridesmaid for Margaret's mother. Our families had met a few times over the course of the years. Indeed, Margaret even lived with us for a short time as a young girl starting work in about 1955/56. As a teenager I thought she was quite beautiful. Margaret, on the other hand, thought I was the typical teenage pest. We did not meet again until 1963.

I had entered the Augustinian Order of priests after finishing high school in 1958. Study towards the priesthood took me to the United States of America. During my years of study I sometimes doubted whether I was on the right track, but persisted until 1963. At that stage I kept wondering how I would react to meeting up with Margaret.

I decided to leave the Augustinian Order and returned to Australia in late 1963. I had no idea whether Margaret was alive or, if alive, whether she was single or married. She was not married. When I first saw her I knew she was the person I wanted to marry. It took Margaret longer to want to spend the rest of her life with me. She did tell me though, that on the day that I had decided to leave my study for the priesthood, she had finished a weekend of prayer and she had an overwhelming sense that something good was to happen to her. We agreed that that was me. We were engaged by the end of 1964 and married in December 1965.

Our married life together, I am sure, was similar to that experienced by many others. There were highs and lows. Our three daughters were definitely highs. Another was Margaret's return to school to complete her senior matriculation and then to graduate from Queensland University with a Bachelor of Arts in 1991.

Margaret was a highly intelligent woman. She was an avid reader. She was a meticulous dressmaker. She loved music and was a member of the Brisbane Girls Choir before our marriage. Her language skills were legend in our family. We all looked to her as our 'dictionary on legs'. Her scholarly and painstaking approach to writing was an example to the girls and me. She consistently received very high marks for her study both at senior and university level. She was introverted by nature, but loved to attend the many functions my occupation required of me. We had the opportunity to travel overseas fairly extensively in the 1990s. She was active in the community through participation in tuck shops, meals on wheels, as well as being reader, Eucharistic minister and visitor to the sick in our local church parish.

By the late 1990s we were at a stage in our lives when we had much to look forward to and enjoy together. With our three daughters grown up and living away from home, or at least we hoped they would be, a new phase of life was about to begin. Retirement from full-time work would allow me to spend time with Margaret pursuing some of our long held dreams. As with many our age, we planned to travel where we wished to go, to play a significant role in the formation of our grandchildren as yet unborn, to be active once more in our local church community, to read and write, to smell the roses together.

Margaret's general health was good. She did suffer from rheumatoid arthritis which was largely kept in check through anti-inflammatory medications. Fortunately that disease limited its attacks to her smaller joints. It did eventually make fine sewing work too difficult for her.

My reason for recording all of this about Margaret is to underscore that with Alzheimer's disease there is no pattern to suggest who will contact it, particularly its early onset. It seems to be no respecter of backgrounds - cultural, educational, emotional or social. Furthermore the early signs that there may be a 'problem' can, for those closest to the sufferer, often be thought to be caused by other things, whatever those things might be. In my own case the use of certain medications to alleviate Margaret's rheumatoid arthritis.

There is, of course, no clearer vision than the 20/20 vision of hindsight. As I look back to the 12 or 18 months period prior to a formal diagnosis of the disease, I can now see soft signs of the disease's progression in Margaret. Perhaps the more obvious sign towards the end of 1997 occurred while I was on a sabbatical break from my job, travelling through parts of Europe and the USA.

We had lived in San Antonio, Texas, for most of 1990 attending University there. Margaret drove everyday on the 'wrong' side of the road without any real trouble, other than the occasional temptation to enter a freeway via an exit route when driving on 'automatic pilot' so to speak. We often thought that we should have a sign - 'Australian at the wheel' - to protect others. However I had a great deal of difficulty coaxing Margaret to drive in the USA in 1997. She found it very confusing to be on the opposite side of the car and road.

In two other areas confusion, I chose to see it as confusion, also reigned. She found it difficult to operate a video camera which we had owned and used over a number of years. She also had great difficulty reading road maps. The road map incidents were really out of character. In fact, I was normally the one who found it difficult to give appropriate directions to the driver. My response to Margaret's confusion was usually to show my arrogance, grab the map and sort it out myself with the typical attitude of, 'what more could you expect from a woman!'

The point I am making here is that for Margaret there were soft signs of something awry. The signs seemed to be evident in dealing with technical changes or any variation from the normal, almost automatic, way of doing things. As well, following or setting out directions to be followed needed time without pressure to be accomplished.

The following year, 1998, was one involving several major events in our lives. I finished my tenure of work in June of that year and at my public farewell Margaret's father died peacefully at his home. I am not suggesting these events had any influence on Margaret's situation. What they did do was give me the time to be at home more often and to observe Margaret's behaviours more closely on a daily basis.

I now became more aware of Margaret's forgetfulness. For example she would now write comprehensive notes about any phone call she took. She was not yet 60 so it could not be 'old age'. I raised the matter with her on 3 August.

"Spoke to Marg about her forgetfulness. She was in tears."

So sensitive was she that I noted I would need to tread warily and be very patient. Only after her death did I find a little notebook in which she had written about an event which took her to the Sunnybank hospital in February of 1998. Had I read that at that time I would have been shocked at the shakiness of her hand and the significant spelling errors. She no doubt was already aware of changes inside herself but was not prepared to share that even with me.

I must emphasise that any thought of dementia never entered my head. I had read somewhere that in some people there could be mental confusion for those who took the drug, Zantac. Margaret had been taking Zantac for years to offset the harsh effects of the anti-inflammatory tablets she took for her rheumatoid arthritis. I harboured a suspicion that this may be at the back of Margaret's confusion and forgetfulness.

I decided to set up my own consultancy business. That took a lot of my time. No wonder then that my journals do not reference Margaret's situation again until 9 November. Her forgetfulness was not life threatening, nor was it disruptive in everyday living. In fact, one could almost see a humorous side to some events. For instance, Margaret had informed our bank that we did not have a pin number for our account. We did of course have one for many years. We now had a new one. I wrote on 9 November:

> *"She is a little weepy these days. I see the hurt in her face and I feel so bad for her. She does have trouble with remembering things."*

I decided to employ Margaret on a part-time basis as my secretary. She had gained some knowledge of computers in her postgraduate course on library work. She had always been a good typist. Though Margaret had the fear of new technology that many people had in our age bracket, she had little trouble in typing and formatting papers for me. Unfortunately the typing aggravated Margaret's arthritis which flared up as the year came to a close.

I realise that my journey with Margaret is at once a very private and personal one, but one by necessity played out in public. In telling our story I struggle between the need to protect our privacy, to respect Margaret's dignity and to provide some support for those presently undertaking a similar journey, or who will do so in the future. This disease does not enjoy the high profile nature of many other illnesses that befall members of our society. It is, however, on the increase. It has devastating effects on the sufferer and the carers, and is a time bomb in terms of its ultimate impact on governments and the community at large.

I have likened the stigma society places on those who suffer from Alzheimer's to that of the leper in Biblical times. It has amazed me how literally terrified so many become by a disease which attacks the brain and thereby affects all the functions of daily living which rely upon the brain for them to be performed in the normal way. The disease cannot be 'caught' from sufferers nor, as far as we know, does the sufferer merit the disease because of their lifestyle. Our experience was that many friends and even extended family members could not deal with the outward expressions seen in the one having the disease. We felt abandoned, outcasts like the lepers of old.

Chapter 2

1999 Testing and Hoping

*T*his year was a seminal year in our journey with Alzheimer's. It did not open that way because our major concern at the outset was the flare up of Margaret's rheumatoid arthritis. We, Margaret together with our youngest daughter Anne and me, had decided to take a short holiday. We flew to Melbourne on 4 January.

The journey was smooth. Margaret was tired after the flight so she had a sleep after lunch. She often liked to lie down after lunch and so I did not consider that there was anything peculiar about her being tired. That evening she delighted in sitting at a sidewalk café in Swanson Street, glad, as we all were, to be spending time together.

When we were out walking Margaret had difficulty with sets of stairs due to her painful rheumatoid arthritis. I had some hope that a new drug, Cerebex, may be good for her. We ventured to Melbourne's casino mainly to watch the parade. Both Margaret and I always found it interesting to study people moving and interacting in public. It was here that I first record Margaret mislaying something. She had put her umbrella down somewhere and it walked. We returned home to warmer weather on 8 January.

It was 17 January when I began to grow more concerned about Margaret's forgetfulness. She had done some ironing and left the iron turned on. That was a real worry for me. It was so out of character for her. I wrote:

> "Don't know what the answer is. I love her so much and hate to see anything change. I only hope it is something simple."

I am sure that at this stage I was in total denial. That mindset would stay with me for many months. I probably could have been more aware of Margaret's changing patterns had I not liked the idea of cooking for example. I now had more time so I did a lot of the cooking, much to Margaret's delight. I also believed I should be more responsible for the heavier house work because of Margaret's arthritis. In the past Margaret would have told me to get out of her kitchen, but now she just accepted my being there and seemed content to help rather than lead. This turned out to be great training for what lay ahead of me. It was February when I was confronted with another soft sign. It did not cross my mind that Margaret feared that she may be embarrassed by forgetting in a public setting. I noted:

> "Out shopping with Margaret. We had words. She can't or won't get used to the credit card system. Has a phobia about it. Wants to write everything down then forgets where."

Her hand writing at this time was rather good. Her hand was steady and the words and spelling were accurate. She did, however, have days during which words she wanted to use when speaking would not come. I remember noting to myself that they tended to be nouns, the names of things or people, rather than verbs. I normally tried to help her recall the word for which she was searching. On 14 February I had made out my first cheque to Margaret as my employee. I asked her to type out an email for me. I had set up the computer so that all she had to do was type out the message.

> "I was really shocked that she seemed to have lost her ability as a typist. She has great problems with spelling also. I know she fears new technology, but this is far more. Wish I knew what to do. I just seem to offend her and I don't mean to do that."

I am unsure whether changes were speeding up within Margaret or I was simply becoming more aware of them. Still, no thought of dementia crossed my mind. I do recall that

Margaret began to experience severe headaches. She had them very occasionally throughout her life, but they were now more frequent and generally severe. One of our daughters had been living away from home for a time. Late in February she told me that she was now much more aware of Margaret's struggle with forgetfulness. I wrote:

> "I live with it and I don't know what to do. I only wish she would have a good check-up. I still think it is largely to do with speech and use of language."

Though I had suggested that Margaret be seen by a physician, she would have none of it. Perhaps, as I reflect, she knew, more so than I did, the struggle she was having and she did not want to know the cause. Fear of the unknown can be very powerful. Ignorance, we convince ourselves, may be bliss.

Although my consultancy work was only getting off the ground, I began to sense that having to spend days away from home was not going to be possible in the future. I must admit that I waxed and waned about this over many months. As early as 10 March I write:

> "I slept soundly until 4am. After that I think I was anxious about leaving Margaret for so long. She was upset I know. I have determined not to let this happen again. There is part of me though that says it may do her good to have to make decisions and do the job. My only real concern generally is at her language skills."

In the light of the future, how inane was my thought that by making her act alone she would improve. Let there be no illusions here. Practice does not stop nor even, in my experience, significantly slow down the inevitable losses that attend the progression of Alzheimer's disease. I was away from home for 10 days. I rang Margaret each night or late each afternoon:

> "I look forward to hearing her voice. All is well on the home front."

Though the next day when I rang:

> "She was not very talkative last night. Just wanted to listen. I miss her so much too."

Margaret drove out to the airport with our youngest daughter Anne to pick me up on my return. Life went on and we enjoyed going out on occasion. I recall we both totally enjoyed seeing a Williamson play, "Corporate Vibes", at the Optus Theatre on 28 April. That evening, however, she had a 'turn'. She got very hot, her face and neck were flushed and she felt giddy.

> "Her eyes showed her concern".

After 10 minutes her temperature returned to normal. I arranged for her doctor to see her later the next day. No abnormality turned up, but I wrote:

> "I am still concerned. I want her to have a good check-up, but she will not go."

It was so unusual for Margaret to have this attitude. She was the one always pushing me and the girls to go to the doctor. Visiting doctors seemed to be a normal event in her life. Nor would this be the last of such episodes or 'turns'. I continued to relate Margaret's state to the possible effects of Zantac. I did struggle, however, with a growing concern that there may be some other cause. My diary entry on 14 May reads:

> "I had a good talk with Margaret during breakfast. She could not subtract 65 from 99. I told her of my deep love for her and how I longed to spend a lot of my allotted life with her. Just this week she could not spell 'sense'. She used to be our walking dictionary."

Our family doctor had mentioned the possibility of having a brain scan. Nothing eventuated unfortunately. By 19 May I wrote:

> "I again found Margaret has lost the most common ability to use numbers. She tries to excuse her inadequacies. I am not

demeaning her but trying to have her realise that she must seek help now. Love her so dearly, this hurts more than I can express."

Whether Margaret's ability with numbers was adversely affected before or after her language, I do not know. Certainly I became aware of that loss after her struggle with words. About June I recognised that Margaret was grinding her teeth at night. I stupidly wrote:

"Wonder too what is worrying her so."

Eventually our family dentist made a small mouth guard which did give her some relief. Margaret did not like using it, so it was later put in a container and left there. Margaret would often snore at night especially when she wore her mouth guard. Her action of 13 July gives an insight into this wonderful person:

"I felt terrible when I found Margaret slept on the couch. She thought that would give me a more peaceful night. It is the epitome of her selfless love. I am so privileged to be her husband. She is so attuned to serving others she does not deserve to be in pain, only to be loved. I pray her arthritis is controlled and that we may have a long and love filled retirement period."

As I look back on such writing I realise that this was the beginning of a reversal of roles for us. I would be called to show selfless love, to serve her needs, to wait upon rather than be waited upon. Such a calling, as I indicated at the outset, can only be premised on a deep and abiding love one for the other.

Margaret was still driving the car. There seemed little reason to be concerned as it was her language use that was suffering. She would often drive me to the airport for example even though I sensed she would rather not have to do so. It must have been quite traumatic for her. Imagine having a degree of concern that you may forget the way home.

My consultancy had me away from home often. That was okay for as long as our daughter, Anne, was at home, but she was off to Japan for a year. I was sure that that would be a major turning point for us. More frequently now as I prepared to head away on business I would note that:

> "Margaret was rather teary about my going. Need to be aware of her needs at the moment."

She never did, however, ask me not to go.

There are many turning points, days to remember as it were, in the Alzheimer's journey. For us one such day was Monday 23 August 1999. My diary best outlines the events as they occurred:

> "Margaret had slept fairly well though I went upstairs at 1am. At 7am Margaret went to the toilet and I thought I could hear her moaning. It grew louder and I grew concerned. Marg was distressed, in panic. She was cold, yet sweating, had tingles in her legs below the knees and also in her hands.
> I rang 000 and had an ambulance come. Then I got Marg into bed. She was very pale and wet and cold. The ambulance came in about 7 or so minutes. They were very good. Gave her oxygen, took a cardiograph then took her to the Mater private. I packed a bag, dressed and went to the Mater by 9am.
> Marg stayed until about 11.30am. They took a cat scan of her lower torso. It showed no abnormalities. Her heart did show some sign of arrhythmia. They thought that she may simply have had a panic or anxiety attack after the heart had fluttered. Marg was not sure."

After I got Margaret home she rested. All she could take was some liquid. She woke at 3.30am the following morning and suffered a less severe attack than that of the day before. I kept talking to her to keep her calm and it worked. Later we went to our family doctor who examined Margaret thoroughly for over 30 minutes. He too believed she may have suffered an anxiety attack. We did though convince Margaret that it was time to see a neurologist and an appointment was made for the following week. Margaret was worn out so slept after a light lunch. By nightfall she seemed far more relaxed.

That night there was a third episode. The nausea and tingling were present, but by being with Margaret and talking to her she eventually went back to sleep. She woke by 6.30am, had a little breakfast and complained of a massive headache. Panadol had no effect but Panadeine did ease it by the end of the day.

Margaret slept well on the fourth night. She looked far more relaxed and her headache had abated. Her appetite was also slowly returning. Throughout this ordeal I don't think I ever really turned my attention to the question of what Margaret may have been anxious about. In hindsight I feel sure she was far more aware than any of us as to the depth of changes occurring in her brain and body.

Monday 30 August came around very quickly. Could I ever forget that day? Could Margaret forget it? Eventually she would forget thank God. We had found our way to Watkins Place by 9.30am. The neurologist seemed to me to be a pleasant enough fellow. Margaret thought that he was abrupt and took a dislike to him which would mellow a little in time. Having asked about her history, he then tested her on names of common items and on listing things like the days of the week backwards. Margaret was very nervous and tense and she did not respond as well as I expected. He determined to do a full program of tests involving a blood test, ceretec scan, MRI and EEG.

> *"Says there is a 10% chance there will be something simple to treat. I got the impression he did not expect that, for he said there was something seriously wrong 'up there'. Will know later after the tests. That shook Marg and myself. I still feel empty in the stomach. I arranged the scan and MRI at the Mater."*

After the consultation we sat at the coffee shop on the ground floor not really wanting to talk. Margaret was in tears and looked very frightened. She still expressed excuses for her poor performance in the doctor's testing. This little routine of coffee after the consultation became part of our way of dealing with what would be an emotionally draining part of our journey.

The next day I was still in shock and was surprised at how deep in the gut was my fear about all that may be revealed through Margaret's tests.

> "I will have to be more balanced. It shows me very clearly how much I love her and how much she is an integral part of myself as I am of her."

September commenced. Let my diary do the talking for me:

> "First day of spring in the autumn of our lives! Today Marg and I look squarely at our mortality. She had her ceretec scan at 7.15 at the Mater and we picked up the results at 3pm. Fortunately or not, we read the report and the world looked so fragile. It talks of significant problems in the frontal and parietal lobes. It suggests possible internal depression, infarctation and /or SDAT, whatever that is (I suspect dementia of one kind or another). We both were in tears. Life sure hangs by a thread and this will test our ability to cope.
> After the Mater I went for a run. I don't pray as I run unfortunately. I was acutely aware of my love for Marg though, how much she is the centre of my being. I thought how beautiful it is to be privileged to experience such love. It is perhaps a glimpse of the all powerful love of God for us."

We spent the rest of the day together and both experienced a bad night.

> "Lord only knows what Marg is feeling. I got an insight into that and her faith when she said out of the blue, 'I wish I were a leper'. Startled, I asked why a leper. She said, 'If I were a leper, He could cure me.' I cried and have been doing so internally a lot."

Life again went on. Margaret looked concerned and pale whenever I was with her. Though I tried always to be supportive of her, I perhaps could have been more attentive to what mental anguish she was suffering. One of the many things I was to learn from our journey was, that at all times, the one having the disease should take centre stage. Often I found myself being more attentive to my own suffering. I know how scared I was about what the future would hold for us. Imagine, just imagine, what it must be like at this point for the sufferer who is intelligent enough to know exactly what may, indeed will, be the outcome.

Although, for now, we were hoping against hope, that there may be a simple explanation.

Father's day was not quite as joyous as had been the case in years past.

> *"It is however coloured by my concern for Margaret's well being and how she is coping. She keeps herself busy I notice. She is quiet yet I know when we are alone how much she is hurting. Even as day ends she tells me of her fear that this time next year she will not be with me."*

Margaret had her MRI on 6 September. We were to see the neurologist on 8 September. Margaret did not want to go, but I talked her into it and said we would assess whether we continued after he had given us his diagnosis. To help take her mind off things she accompanied me on a consultancy job at Toowoomba. She enjoyed the day.

I think my diary entry for Wednesday 8 September sums up best our visit to the neurologist.

> *"If 27 July 1996 was a D day - dark that is - for me when I had a heart attack, in many ways this was one for Margaret. We have been living in fear about seeing the doctor today.*
> *We left for the Terrace at 1.30. At 2.15 Marg had an EEG, then we saw the doctor at 3.10. He was very nice. Margaret even liked him. He was more humane and caring. He had all test results. The scan and EEG showed areas of inactivity. The MRI showed no growths or bleeds thank God. The doctors did not note any abnormalities but the neurologist disagrees. He thinks the cells of the brain are dying and it is shrinking in places. The blood test shows Marg needs B-12 supplements and her thyroid is not as active as it should be. Wants to treat those first. If that works - OK. If not then it is his view that this is the onset of Alzheimer's. That is a death sentence of how long we do not know. What I do know is that we have been much blest in this life and that we must face the future bravely together. I do know that miracles are possible so I put my trust in God. Should God have other plans I hope we have the grace to deal with them too. Meantime we must get on with life and living. The*

> *girls all rang and were upset. They are our three most precious blessings together with their friends, partners and, we hope, children. Mary with your loving Son your blessing give to us all this day."*

We placed our hope in the success of the B-12 and thyroid treatments. I now bought and read several books on Alzheimer's disease and read articles taken from the internet. Margaret too read these. Every change or inability to do simple things took on greater significance. I allowed myself to grow annoyed at times, with no justification other than I so desperately wanted Margaret to get better. When she could not remember dates or use our new can opener, it would inevitably lead to tears and frustration for us both.

I kept on with my consultancy. Margaret seemed to cope at home by herself despite my growing concerns. She travelled to Rockhampton with her mother to spend some time with me and our very close friends. We had a weekend at Yeppoon.

> *"I realised again today how much I love my Margaret. She will require my close attention and I do not know if I am capable of all that my God will ask of me. What a privilege it has been to have had her as my wife for so long."*

Because we still had hopes of a miracle, we let no one know how serious Margaret's condition may be other than sharing it with our daughters. In public it was still reasonably easy to cover over any forgetfulness by Margaret.

We had a golf day while at Yeppoon. Margaret enjoyed it. She could not play, not that I could all that well either, but she drove the golf buggy around for me. It did me good to have her enjoy herself so much.

I invited Margaret to go walking with me. I had assumed that she would not enjoy it in the past. How wrong I was. Walking together was to become a regular event for us in the years ahead. We stopped only when she could no longer walk unaided.

Often as I write I am reminded that a good friend of mine, Marcel, once told me that this life is not a dress rehearsal, so we need to enjoy life as it is dealt to us. One of my regrets was not heeding that advice. When you accept that a disease cannot be cured, when it sets even an unknown but certain limit to a lifespan, take all the opportunities that are presented to enjoy life. Make good and happy times happen. The sad times will take care of themselves and you will have no control over their coming.

During late October Margaret had another of her 'turns'. My diary indicates how frequent these were at this point in our journey. Margaret usually turned an ashen colour, lost her appetite and always felt a 'discomfort' in the head. Her language skills were already rapidly deteriorating and, coupled with the anxiety of feeling unwell, it was difficult for her to articulate clearly how she felt and what she wanted to do. These 'turns' would have an effect on her for days at a time.

Doubts about my being able to effectively continue to work were with me daily. Especially when she was unwell, I could see that Margaret had to be given most of my attention. She never asked for that, but I knew how much more at ease she was when I could focus totally on her and her needs. I found myself feeling depressed at times about this. Could I cope with what lay ahead? Did I have sufficient financial backing to provide for us adequately, etc? As I noted in November:

> *"I packed. Margaret had heart flutters early in the morning. It was hard to leave her. She is not confident at all. I have a real decision to make about continuing to work. Boy I love her though."*

I think in everyone's journey with Alzheimer's there will be the inevitable loss of keys story. Ours occurred on 6 November. Margaret had been home all day but for a short journey to the corner store. Her set of keys had disappeared. We were sure they were in the house somewhere if only they could be found. We searched high and low and I wondered about changing the locks. Two days later Margaret found them. They were on one of the lounge chairs covered by the cushions. How we had missed them in our searching I don't know. Margaret's joy was truly of biblical proportions. It reminded me of the widow's mite story in the Bible. The widow had searched her whole house before she finally found the money she had lost and her joy was great because she had so little.

As more people heard about Margaret's potential illness, we experienced a number of disconcerting behaviours on their part. In some cases one was given the feeling that Margaret was now some sort of imbecile who could not understand what was being said about her, even when it was said in her presence. In fact Margaret was still coping well generally, even driving the car, doing the washing and going shopping as well as caring for all her personal needs. It was as if once the dreaded 'A' word was used, the sufferer became incapable of understanding and full participation. This hurt Margaret deeply although she was too much of a lady to let it be shown publicly.

It is difficult enough to cope with all the effects of this disease without others automatically assuming the sufferer is somehow intellectually impaired. I cannot stress this enough. Margaret was not suffering from a loss of intelligence. Alzheimer's attacks the brain so that the sufferer cannot operate in the way they normally would. The messages from the brain simply get scrambled and cannot find their way to wherever the sufferer would normally direct them. You need friends and family to fully understand this and always treat the person with respect and dignity, giving them the benefit of any doubt about their level of understanding, even if they cannot clearly communicate verbally that they do understand.

Over the weeks the B-12 supplements raised Margaret's B-12 to the normal range. Still her memory was problematic. Meanwhile, she developed some arthritis in her neck that required physiotherapy. That gave her some relief.

My eldest sister passed into eternity in November. Her funeral was held on 23 November. The family nature of the ceremony made it very special we thought. Margaret and I had been special ministers in our church so we were invited to help distribute communion from the altar. My beautiful Margaret was both delighted and wary. I noticed how confused she became. I quietly explained to her what to do and she did it. This was to be the last time she would so participate. It was also the beginning of a period of my having to be watchful so as to help her and not allow her to be publicly embarrassed.

We would visit the neurologist one more time in 1999. Margaret began to grow anxious about that day even before it was due. I note on 6 December:

> "Soon after rising she got a wave of hot and 'funny' feelings from her gut up. We talked about fear, stress, etc. Seemed OK then it happened at 9am. Thought she would not go. I talked her into keeping the appointment. Got to see the Dr at 10.20. He was rather nice. Tested her again. Said she seemed no worse. I believe that, but there are worse times than others."

Later in the day Margaret had another 'turn'. I took her to our family doctor, but he too thought it was due to stress. For both of us going to see the neurologist was a trip simply to hear more bad news. Margaret was never going to hear that her disease was cured and she knew that to be the case. As the year closed Margaret's disease was having an effect on me also.

> "There are times I get so frustrated with Marg and I have no right to. She would not drive Anne into town by herself. She is losing confidence. She seldom takes an initiative to prepare a meal. She went to the chemist and was embarrassed by not knowing the date. It goes on and on. I wonder what the future holds for us. I am not the most patient of carers. She has cared for me this past 30 plus years. I am not sure I am made of the stuff required to look after her."

As yet I had no clear idea what it would take to be her carer. I would find out.

Chapter 3

2000

Towards Fulltime Caring

As a child I was deeply affected by the story of Jesus curing the ten lepers and His disappointment that only one returned to thank Him. Prayer had always been integrated into my daily life, though some days I was far more prayerful than on others. I had been brought up, as indeed had my generation of Roman Catholics, on a diet of prayer to Mary the Mother of God. In particular praying the rosary was an essential component. Over the years that prayer became less frequent, but I am not too proud to admit to finding it again. As I wrote on 3 January:

> *"I have formed a habit of saying the rosary as I walk. I find it refreshing and I can pray for all the family as well as give thanks. I particularly talk to God about my beautiful Margaret."*

For carers who have a religious belief I cannot stress enough the value of prayer. It may not seem to be answered. In my case asking for a miracle cure fell on deaf ears. Instead I think, in fact I know, I received help in ways I could not have imagined. The miracle was that I was able to look after Margaret all the time that this disease went on its inexorable course.

As I began to notice more little changes in Margaret's behaviour, I would react at times like a bear with a sore head. I was both frustrated and saddened to see that her forgetfulness ranged way beyond words and numbers. She would leave doors and drawers open, empty the rubbish basket but forget to bring it back with her. When I would point these things out to her she would become very upset.

Margaret was quite capable of carrying on an intelligent conversation with visitors. She could do the laundry without difficulty, but:

> "She had not cooked a meal for over three months. She will find any excuse not to have to prepare tea."

The internal struggle I was having about whether to continue with my consultancy work or to give it away was a major component of my intemperate reactions at times. Tiredness was also a significant factor in retaining control of my own emotions.

I had tried to coax Margaret into writing a diary. I thought that it may assist her to retain the use of language. Try as I might, she would refuse to do so. I can now understand that. It would have been a constant and concrete reminder to her of the loss of competencies she was experiencing. I mention this because it helps me to realise that often my suggestions did not consider matters from her perspective. On many, many occasions this was so. I think it behoves the carer to try to walk in the sufferer's shoes, to see things through his or her eyes. I would have been far less judgemental and hopefully more patient if I had done so.

Margaret's headaches continued. Even at this early stage it was difficult for me to address her needs as she would struggle for the right words to explain just what was happening. How tragic for a woman who crafted her word usage, and who more often than not got 19 or 20 out of 20 for her written university assignments in literature. Margaret had received a letter from the Head of the Department of English on 12 January 1988. Amongst other things it read:

> "Your ability to attain this standard suggests that you should seriously consider the possibility of taking English Honours Fourth Year at the conclusion of your pass course."

On 26 January 2000:

> *"I sat Marg down at the computer. She had some time on the internet. Looked at some info on Alzheimer's. Did not make her happy. She gets depressed about it all. Later got her to send a short email to Anne. It was painful to watch her type. The skill which was once so well developed is now very hard for her. She felt it too I am sure. I love her so much it is not funny. We must remain positive though and enjoy our lives. I cooked tea and then we relaxed for the evening."*

By 10 February my diary note gives some indication of the speed of change that Margaret was undergoing:

> *"She was in tears this morning. Tried writing down months of the year and then backwards. Found that even too hard. She does not understand, why her. She is tormented all the time as words will not flow. My prayers go unanswered seemingly. I try to convince her that though we may/will fail, we should fight it - use the mind continuously."*

We grew to be interested in any article about research into Alzheimer's. We wished that it had a public profile like AIDS, with money made available for research in such areas. It was all about clutching at straws of hope. Eventually I knew that even any breakthrough would come too late to be of help for Margaret. Hope is one of the most powerful of forces in our lives. When it is taken away, ones will and strength are sorely tested.

I noticed one day how much Margaret's eyes told me. She looked so very lonely and I wondered what life would be like for her if I were not at home most of the time. Her difficulty with language, especially nouns, seemed to grow very quickly. I would make her use the correct words but:

> *"It is like being a young child again and it really disturbs her."*

The image of the young child was not really apt as the young child usually learns and matures. My Margaret was regressing steadily, not progressing.

We had a visit to the neurologist planned for 6 March. The day before the visit Margaret was in tears. Just the thought of going to see him disturbed her:

> "She does not want to be as she is. I am not as good a support as I should be. I still hope and pray for a cure. God give us both strength and faith."

As it turned out the visit was simply to help the doctor ascertain the speed of the disease's progression. He asked us to return in six months. Of the disease:

> "I must admit at times I think it is worse than I think. Her ability to listen to and follow instructions is poor, and common things – like how to use a calendar – she claims were never before explained to her. We have a pact to try to live life and enjoy it."

Our pact was developed as we sat in the cafe drinking our coffee at Watkins Place that morning. We decided, therefore, to go for a trip overseas. I thought it would be our last trip and I wanted it to be at a time when Margaret could enjoy the experience. We planned to begin our journey in September.

My inner conflict about continuing to work flared up more often. I can imagine this is a potential problem for anyone whose life role has been to work to provide for the family. In our married life I had always been the sole income earner. Margaret's chosen workplace was the home for the family. On 11 March I wrote:

> "Have been feeling low today. I think I know I should give up my consultancy to look after/be with Marg and I don't want to do so. It is a sense of failure in my life. Sounds stupid but it is there. I watch and listen. Her language use is growing worse. I am embarrassing her too at times by demanding she use the right words. I am not good at this caring caper. I also wonder how I will cope with nothing of substance to do. It really frightens me."

How strange it is for me to read that I could have thought the role of carer lacked substance. It was my experience that no other occupation I had had demanded so much of me. Our daily grind continued and Margaret struggled to come to terms with her disease.

> "I helped Marg to read the calendar again. We both got upset. She keeps wondering how long she has before she dies and I weep because I see her pain. 'I don't want this to be happening to me', she says in tears. It is a very hard time for us. I must support her, I pray for a miracle, I feel lost not working and so the cycle goes. She is looking so thin. I love her more than life itself and often cry by myself when she cannot see me."

We had a couple of short trips away from home which we both greatly enjoyed. At times Margaret would get annoyed with me for talking to any other person about her disease. Even when I told her that our family doctor had asked after her she cried.

> "Hates to hear that she may be getting worse, but the reality is that slowly she is."

As fate would have it on this night we watched a TV program called 'ER'. It centred upon a doctor with Alzheimer's disease. We determined to use that experience.

> "We must be able to discuss it ourselves naturally or we will have a very unhappy few years."

We also agreed to keep it as much as possible within the family. There was an election on 25 March. I had a difficult time explaining the system to Margaret. This was a real eye opener for me. Margaret had always loved election time and would sit and watch the outcome on TV for both State and Federal elections. For the first time it came home to me that Margaret may eventually be unable to cope with most aspects of normal life.

Our first grandchild arrived on March 27. Margaret adored her little granddaughter, named Emer. She had great difficulty in trying to learn a new name. Initially she would feign not having been told. I guess she really believed that as she simply could not recall it. With persistent practice though, she did come to recognise the name. She had no difficulty recognising the face.

Years later I was given a set of video tapes compiled by the BBC on the nature of the brain. Much of it I cannot recall, but one feature I noted because I saw it so often in action. If I am correct, it seems that a particular part of the brain helps us recognise faces and is separate from most other functions of recognition. It is good to keep this in mind as a carer. If the component of the brain set aside for the recognition of faces remains relatively unaffected by the disease, the sufferer will recognise the face long after the loss of names. Margaret recognised faces to the day she died.

Forgetfulness was of growing concern. We went to see the movie, "The Green Mile" in April. It was long but Margaret enjoyed the outing. She went to the rest room on the way out and left her purse there. It had walked by the time she became aware that she did not have it. Luckily a woman, Denise, rang to say she found the purse in the street. The cash had gone, but all Margaret's cards were safe. We gave Denise a bottle of wine and two lottery tickets in thanks. The next day I had asked Margaret to put on some corned beef to cook while I was out. At one stage I guess Margaret took the lid off the saucepan, left it on the gas stove and the handle burned off. Poor darling had a burnt hand when I got home.

Though Margaret was still doing the weekly washing by herself and the ironing, I worried about how she would cope during our planned trip to Canada in September. As well, I suspected that we were reaching a point where Margaret should no longer drive the car. Our overseas trip would entail a significant amount of driving.

To try to assist Margaret to use names effectively, I began having a game with her. We would walk through the house and she would try to name the rooms and/or the furniture therein. She did well for a time. I had to approach this as a game or it became too stressful for her. It took a lot of coaxing. She was smart enough to guess what I was up to.

Answering the phone was problematic. When Margaret was talking to a family member it progressed reasonably. If it was someone other than family, she would grow confused and even hang up in mid conversation. I would have to concoct a story that our line just dropped out. At other times we would not be contactable because Margaret would simply put the phone down wherever she happened to be when she was finished with her conversation. Thank God we had a signal to help locate the handset.

Throughout this whole period, I note in my diaries that Margaret regularly has what I call a 'turn'. These were not as violent as the one's I have already described that occurred in 1999. On 29 April:

> "Margaret was not feeling well. Told me she had one of her 'turns' last night, but did not mention it to me. Seems she had a cold, chill feeling travel down her arms and her tummy feels funny. Sometimes she feels things are not OK in her head also. She is not clear, in fact very muddled when trying to tell me. Only by patient questioning can I get somewhere."

And again a month later on 30 May:

> "Margaret woke feeling crook. Had one of her turns later. Looks ashen and her eyes show fear. Tells me she has a feeling that begins in her head and passes down through her body, like a wave. It is hard to decipher exactly as she gets confused at these times. I feel inadequate to deal with it."

Life had become a real roller coaster ride. We shared in the joy of Margaret preparing tea for the first time in months, with just a little help from me. She drove the car home from the grocery store on my insistence. I knew that left to herself she would not drive. However, after attending a seminar around tea time, I returned home to find that Margaret had not been able to follow the instructions I had left. She had eaten nothing:

> "She is now little capable of looking after herself as far as food is concerned. I got annoyed more at myself for leaving her. She was upset as I think she knows this shows how dependant she's becoming."

Sometime later:

> "We had traveller's cheques to pick up at the Bank of Qld. I had them all in Margaret's name. She had to sign them all. She panicked as the woman watched her and twice could not spell O'Rourke. I had to coach her. She was embarrassed and I was a little shocked. She will now practice as I have been asking her."

The more complex the task the more difficult did Margaret find it. Even taking her medication in different ways and at different times caused concern. Her difficulty in signing her own name caused her the most stress. Indeed, on 7 June, after a similar incident, she told me she would rather die than be as she is. By the end of June I decided to stop work to give my total attention to my Margaret's needs. That decision followed upon one of my trips away from home without her.

> "Most of the morning was set to my packing. Had fun trying to find the books on Alzheimer's we had bought. Marg had hidden them in one of the clothes drawers. I was so distressed at leaving her at home. She too looked as if I was abandoning her. I have determined I will not do this again. Megan will look after her."

I actually felt better within myself after this decision. It was time for me to change roles as I noted on the evening of 1 July:

> "Marg is in bed asleep. She was a bit confused at times today. I so love her. Her life has been one of total service to all of us, especially me."

The change from my work life was not smooth. I believe giving up work actually added to my moodiness:

> "I was in a bad mood in the evening. Some days I get tired of it all. What a selfish attitude. I am close to tears often too. That can't be good for one."

Our neurologist had given us some indication that the disease in Margaret's case was moving quickly and so we should get certain things in place sooner rather than later. So in July we met with our solicitor to begin the process of renewal of wills and preparing powers of attorney. It was essential that such powers related to matters of health as well as our finances. The process was completed by the end of July. Margaret was excellent about it all. We had always had a will and we had been through the process of developing powers of attorney years earlier when we travelled overseas. Her main concern was that she may not be able to complete her signature. She did sign all documents very well. Early attention to updating wills and powers of attorney is extremely important in everyone's journey with such a debilitating disease.

Activities which Margaret had carried out for the entirety of our married lives grew to be so difficult for her. I have mentioned that Margaret did the weekly washing and enjoyed doing that. Nevertheless, on 17 July she could not figure out how to program the washing machine. In a relatively short time her skills in every aspect of life would be stripped from her little by little. How devastating this must have been for her. It was difficult enough for me to observe let alone try to help her retain each skill for as long as possible.

Our family doctor had the point of view that exercising the brain would slow the progression of the disease. The neurologist did not necessarily agree. No matter how often we were to practice skills, they all faded such that even the practice became an emotionally draining exercise. I have kept some sheets of paper of Margaret's signatures she practised writing each day. Eventually she could only manage to write MMO. She just could not recall what came after that. At one point I thought of changing her signature to MMO, but then realised even that would go in due time.

When the time approached to visit the neurologist again, Margaret was upset as usual. She would have me go over with her the type of tests he would carry out on her memory. We would even continue this while driving to the doctor's surgery. I could not convince Margaret that her loss of short term memory was not a reflection of her level of intelligence.

Throughout this period we never lost our hope for a miracle cure. A news report from an Alzheimer's Conference in Washington about a new drug AN17-92 by a doctor Dale Shank which showed promise on mice gave us renewed hope. The hope soon subsided and reality took over again. I realised the time lapse between effectiveness on mice and effectiveness for mankind far exceeded the timeline I understood to be available for Margaret.

When Margaret was tested by the neurologist, she could answer none of his questions correctly. She could not even recall his name or the day of the week despite the fact we had practised these responses on the journey to see him. He wanted to see us again in November and called for more tests and scans before wishing us well on our overseas trip. I could see that his eyes were telling me that I was biting off a fair amount of work for myself.

Before that trip we had a wedding. Our second daughter, Megan, was married on 2 September. We bought Margaret a beautiful red suit to wear. She looked so stunning in it. The wedding went very smoothly and Margaret enjoyed it very much. It is only now that I realise that the next time Margaret wore that outfit was to her own funeral. By 5 September:

> *"Margaret and I spent the day sorting out what we were to take on our trip. That was a feat. Good old Marg keeps trying on the clothes I put out, or taking them elsewhere in the house. I really had fun trying to keep her on track."*

Our trip lasted from 6 September to 15 October. We hired a car in Los Angeles and drove some 12000 kilometres. We travelled up the West Coast to Canada, toured the Rockies, then through Idaho and part of Montana to Wyoming. From there we drove through South Dakota, Nebraska, Colorado, Kansas, Missouri, Arkansas and on to Texas. Naturally we stayed at various places along the way. Margaret did none of the driving. She would wake every night in a different room wondering where we were. Still she seemed to love the scenery and only once on the journey did she have one of her 'turns'.

Our only major mishap was an accident on a country road in Kansas. No other car was involved. It did leave Margaret rather shaken for several days. In all, the exercise was well worth the effort. It was the driving that took its toll on me. This would prove to be our final long vacation together. Travelling by car had allowed us to have many meaningful discussions, another ability soon to be lost. For a time our minds were distracted from the disease she suffered. On our first full day back home, 18 October, I note:

> "During the morning my beautiful wife had to ask me how to make a cup of coffee. I could have cried, but I know she is trying and must find it so hard to have to ask these things."

While we were on our trip we had our meals provided for us. If Margaret could not regularly repeat an action it would be all the more quickly lost.

When I grew tired or was not feeling well myself, I would snap at Margaret for her little lapses. We would then sit and talk, sometimes cry together. She would tell me she is trying, but finds it all very hard. I would apologise and feel guilty for having been short with her. It was becoming more obvious that she could not cope alone. It was not helping our situation that I was having some medical tests carried out also. I kept Margaret in the dark. I was worried about what would happen if I were not around to care for her. Fortunately my tests relieved me of the spectre of cancer.

Margaret had another 'turn' at the end of October. I took her to see our family doctor. He was of the opinion that it was somehow connected to Margaret's Alzheimer's. During the visit I noticed how annoyed Margaret grew because we talked about her rather than to her. That was a great learning for me. Although she was unable to express it in so many words, she was in effect saying, "For God's sake I am right here. Don't treat me as if I am invisible and, even worse, unintelligent". Early in November:

> "Got Margaret to sit with me for almost an hour in the morning. We listed colours, wrote them, then tried to recall them. Want to do this a few times a week to use her brain. Her short term memory is weak as too is her ability to concentrate. Spelling and writing are getting worse too. She can have trouble reading but generally manages quite well."

Sometimes Margaret would get very upset at her inabilities. She knew only too well how her language and mathematic skills had faded. Our daughters noted how much time she was now spending in the bedroom rearranging items. I guess it gave her something to do. At times there appeared to be no rhyme or reason to the level of her confusion. She got confused about how to control the hot water tap at the kitchen sink, yet had no trouble getting herself a drink of cold water or mixing cold and hot to have her shower. As well Margaret began to interpret instructions for action very literally.

As usual, the day before our next visit to the neurologist saw Margaret grow very anxious. We would again prepare as if she were going to sit an exam.

> "After tea Marg sat upstairs 'studying' for her visit to the doctor. This was of little use. She could not remember. Tears flow and somehow I try to help us make sense of this cross. God knows we must learn to enjoy the life we are given. She knows worse lies ahead."

The neurologist asked Margaret about her holiday. He asked me what I had experienced so I talked about her trouble with words and following instructions. He determined that Margaret should have another EEG and a brain scan to see what is happening. Of course there is no cure in sight. He advised that Margaret should no longer drive. I was pleased about that as I was having my own doubts about her being able to make the right decisions in any emergency. Some two days later Margaret was not feeling well. I wrote:

> "Has a far away look. Asked her to do some reading. She says OK but then does not do any. I can't fathom her not wanting to do everything to slow up her mental deterioration."

It was not until some time later that I saw how difficult reading was for her. Throughout her life Margaret had been an avid and fast reader. Early in December I got a great pre-Christmas gift, one that helped me feel inwardly at peace. I met with my middle daughter, Megan, who had married Ben in September:

> "We talked a bit about Marg and where the disease was at. Megan says whatever happened to me she would look after mum even if

it meant she had to give up work. I was inwardly delighted, but please God I will be able to care for my beautiful wife."

At times when we were out shopping, Margaret would look lost. She confided in me that she actually feels lost and is not far from tears all the time. Though I ask her to write about her experiences, I sense it is already too late for that. She is far more at ease rearranging items on and in the tallboy.

It surprises me to read in my diary that at this early stage in my role as carer I would have days when I felt very low. I had one or two jobs from my consultancy business that needed completion before I could totally close it off. The tone of my entry of 6 December gives some sense of my frustrations, let alone Margaret's.

"I watched Marg today. She says she has nothing to do. I point to things but she does not want to do them. Left alone she will head into the bedroom to rearrange a drawer or the contents of her purse. I need to get her to sign a document for tax and that was an effort. I plead with her to write every day but she does not. When the phone rang during breakfast she could/would not get her own toast, etc. Simple enough tasks are becoming hard for her. I can feel myself crying within. I see the pain in her eyes. I am not a good nurse."

Doing the laundry was still Margaret's main job. She enjoyed it once I got the machine set up for her. We had a regular confrontation though when I would try to get her to wash her own clothes. She simply did not want to put her clothes in the wash for whatever the reason. This was quite removed from her normal behaviour. I could also get her to iron shirts for me as long as I stayed around and talked with her. In doing this I could then ensure that the iron was turned off when she had finished. Of course due to her forgetfulness there was the odd accident to contend with. Margaret forgot to turn off the tap in the kitchen and as the sink plug was in we had a little flooding. My difficulty was in seeing the funny side of such events at the time.

As the year came to an end there was one delightful happening. Prior to Christmas our church had a second rite of reconciliation. We, about 100 parishioners, prayed together then examined our consciences to privately enumerate our sins against God. Next we were to go up to one of four priests to confess and seek forgiveness. Margaret got totally confused with the process, so I went up to the priest with her. For the first and only time in my life I had to confess my faults before God, a priest and my wife. It may have been the only time I was pleased my wife suffered from short term memory loss.

Chapter 4

2001

Towards Total Reliance

I find references to Margaret continuing to experience her 'turns' for the months of January, February, June and December in my 2001 diary. Such episodes may not be common to most Alzheimer sufferers. I saw this as a special cross for my Margaret, one that she would have to bear throughout the course of her disease. The first of her 'turns' for this year occurred on 10 January:

> *"I went for a walk. Marg did not want to come. Turned out later in the morning she was having one of her 'funny turns'. She looked pale. She gets very anxious about it too. Spent most of the day resting. Even at night as I was preparing tea she suddenly felt bad. Her poor language skills makes it difficult for me to know what is going on. It seems that a wave goes over her. She never is physically ill, but has a sense of a headache coming."*

Margaret was affected for four days following this 'turn'. Her eyes were very lifeless throughout. When she began to suffer similarly on 12 February I wrote:

> *"She was excellent in her approach to it. She said she would not lie down and would not give in."*

It was great at such times to see her fighting spirit. To squarely face adversity was much more in tune with her character as I had come to know it over the years.

Margaret had a number of smaller episodes, but it is not until 7 June that I again note:

> "About 6.15am Margaret went to the toilet, came back to bed and then had a panic attack. Her right leg kept jumping and her breathing was shallow and sharp. She was wet in the palms also. She had a pain near the lobe of her right ear and later talked of a sore left arm. I did not know what to do. I try to remain calm but she is unable to tell me exactly what is going on. She seems to hallucinate also."

By late afternoon Margaret was in really good form again. I observed that following a significant 'turn' she would become a little more confused.

Margaret began to look for other people in the house and even in the car at times. This was especially evident after her daughters had visited. She seemed to think that they had not gone to their respective homes but were somewhere in the house. From this point in our journey her attempts at conversation were almost impossible to follow. I knew she had something to say to me or to others, but she could not match the words to her thoughts. She had entered what I lovingly like to think of as her 'fruit salad' conversational period.

> "Marg has been a little vague today at times. She wants to join in at other times, but what she has to say has little relevance to the conversation. At least that is what I hear. She, on the other hand, seems to see relevance."

Good and faithful friends are a huge blessing. On 22 November we had a fine meal with Leo and Lyn who have been dear friends for years.

> "Marg feels comfortable with them and enjoyed it. I try not to get embarrassed by some of her wanderings – she tries to participate in conversation, at times well, at other times with

no real relevance to the conversation going on. I guess there is seldom a day when I could not cry as I watch the slow deterioration. I pray for a miracle but expect little. Maybe that is why none comes. What type of faith do I truly have? Still amongst the sadness is always a moment of joy, smiles and certainly great love."

The progression of Margaret's disease and accompanying deterioration is given much space in my diary for 2001. Margaret had always loved reading. Since reading was so important a part of her life, I would sit with her and we would read together. I record on 31 January:

"I sat down with Margaret for almost an hour and we read to one another. Guess I did not know how far her reading skills had deteriorated. I am determined we must do these exercises each day. She knows too that she must exercise her brain. Her writing is not good either. Can well understand why she does none now."

Strangely, Margaret could still spell reasonably well those words she could recall. The writing of them was another issue. Words would just not flow from her pen. Her motor skills were being destroyed. We continued regularly with the reading. As time went on it became more my reading to her than her reading. As well her attention span grew shorter so that our hour sessions became 15 – 20 minutes at most. I felt as if I was teaching a small child how to form words verbally, though in Margaret's case the skill deteriorated despite our practice.

I was particularly keen to ensure, as mentioned earlier, that Margaret could sign her own name for as long as possible. It was, I observed, one of those activities that meant so much to her. Once I tried to mix signature practice with the writing of numbers. It was a disaster. When her brain was attuned to a particular activity it was nigh impossible to immediately switch to another. This is my record of 5 March:

"Marg and I spent some time with her writing her signature. So strange to watch her do it ten times, then when I ask her

> *to count to 10 she does so easily. Writing is a different matter. Her mind is tuned in to the signature. She tries to write the numbers but her signature is the result. I cover the signature and then she can do 1-10. That is about her limit. In numbers and in other writing she has regressed greatly in a relatively short period of time."*

Later in the month our second daughter, Megan, had her birthday. Margaret and I talked about it and our memories of her 32 years as our child. Sadly most of the wonderful memories were lost to Margaret already. I found that it helped her to remember events by looking at old photographs. Margaret would, however, become

> *"So disappointed because she knows she cannot remember."*

On 4 April a female police officer came to the front door. Margaret answered. It appeared that someone had broken into the home next door. By the time I got to the door Margaret had informed the officer that her name was Margaret Clarke. Clarke was her maiden name. It surprised me and hurt a little to have to correct this. A day earlier I had written a fuller account of the deterioration that was now evident.

> *"Marg has had a funny day. I am not sure what has happened in her mind but she has been 'confused'. Talks of the 'others' and 'people'. I think she has some belief that others – our kids – are still at home. Wonders whether some of her clothes are really hers and asks why we should be looking after others' clothes. I went out to tennis in the afternoon and was away from 3.15 to 6.15. She really misses my company. I am always in two minds what to do - to go out regularly or to stay at home. I find my heart crying out at her plight secretly, almost daily, and often many times in the day. I am frightened of the times ahead yet try to concentrate on enjoying this time. I wonder what she will do if I am injured or taken sick while away from her. I pray that my health will be good – physical and mental – so I can truly care for her.*
> *She is the love of my life, of that there is no doubt. I just get dirty with everyone - God included - that she should so suffer. It*

is a suffering not as overt as cancer and the like, but insidious. What makes her human – her memory and use of language - is being taken from her and there is nothing we can do. Prayer seems to be ineffectual. I bang on the door but it seems to remain shut. She spends so much time in the bedroom and rearranging the stuff in her drawers. Once tidy she cannot easily find where things are. I love her and I hope deeply that there is happiness and joy somewhere for us both."

To ensure there was some variety in our existence we had several holidays during the year. In April we went to Norfolk Island with close friends - Marcel and Cath, Ian and Gail. There were always going to be problems. When it came to filling out the customs forms we struck trouble.

"Asked Marg to sign, she got halfway then lost it. She tried to practise but got worse rather than better. I finally told her to leave it alone. She was shaking all over - could not get a cup to her mouth. I put a rug around her and we sat together until she calmed down."

This was a trip to remember for a host of reasons. Our first venture to the airport in Brisbane saw us arriving only to be later sent home. The weather was too bad to allow for a safe landing on the island. Three days later on 26 April it was all systems go. I had thought that Margaret may never sign anything again, but even with our friends looking on Margaret signed her name without a hitch. She had to do so twice more and never flinched. The few days on the island were most enjoyable for us both. The only issue was Margaret's growing very agitated while out with Cath and Gail on a shopping excursion. It was alleviated by simply taking her back to her room.

In May we drove to Rockhampton, about an eight hour car journey. Margaret's elderly mother accompanied us. As we had experienced when we were in the United States, Margaret found it hard to adapt to changed environments. She did however enjoy the journey and the couple of outings we had. Later in July we travelled with friends to Yeppoon on the central coast. It was a golfing weekend. Margaret did not play but enjoyed being out in the open air and driving the golf buggy for me.

Our final trip for the year was to visit Longreach in Central Queensland. I was born there. I had often promised to take Margaret to see my birth place. I thought it was a case of now or never. She liked the car travel as long as we had frequent stops to see the towns and have the traditional cuppa. She was confused by the different motel rooms. They were not her home. It was obvious how much her sense of security was tied into being in her own home environment. One of my diary notes about the journey reads:

> "At one stage Marg looked in the back seat of the car and was surprised no one was with us. Has a mindset that the girls are with us. I knew that she would be disoriented but not quite as much. Have to keep telling her where we are going, why etc. When it looked like rain at one stage she suggested we head home. Distance is a foreign concept now. Still she was interested in all that happened."

It was now necessary to take others into our confidence about Margaret's condition. This was especially so when we were to share a meal with others. I was pleased that I did so with my dear cousin whom we visited while in Longreach. It helped Esma to understand Margaret's action at tea that evening when she tried to eat the apple crumble and custard with her fork. It also made it so much easier for me to direct Margaret in the more appropriate way to act which I would do with as little fanfare as possible to save her any embarrassment. For her part my darling wife would mix in with the conversations being held, even though what she had to say usually had little relevance to the topic at hand. It takes caring and patient people to go with the flow and make the sufferer feel 'normal'. It is a simple way to help ensure that someone like Margaret is always treated with dignity.

This was a year in which there would be changes in a whole range of normal activities. It was truly a sign of things to come in the years ahead. Dressing for example was an area where difficulties were now encountered.

> "I have noticed a further deterioration in Margaret over the past week. Language skills slip a little each week and I have come to

> *partly expect that. Now it is applying to not so complex matters such as dressing. Much has to do with choice. Trying to decide what to wear takes time. Then there is where to wear it. If she is not thinking, she can put on two singlets, one over the other, then gets embarrassed by what she has done. I am tending to help her decide then walk away only to check her out later. She is close to tears at times and it cuts me up to watch her."*

That was in April. If I did not approach her sensitively she would get annoyed with me. I now realise that to dress oneself does indeed involve a number of complex, interrelated activities. Difficulty with dressing led to a number of humorous incidents. At times we both had a laugh, but more generally such incidents were hurtful for my beautiful wife. For example, one morning Margaret came out to breakfast asking if I could help her find her second sock. We began to look around then I noticed that she had put two socks on the one foot.

I try to capture some of the sensitivity surrounding Margaret's dressing of her self on 28 May:

> *"Marg has real problems with some of her dressing in the mornings. Other times there is no problem. She is upset, or was so, that I may think she can no longer dress herself. I am unsure how to act at times. I try to be helpful but I think I come across as telling her what to wear."*

As time went on I would have to dress her. For now it was enough to help set out what to wear and know the process would take a long time. I certainly could not rush Margaret. Dressing herself was only a problem for Margaret in the mornings.

> *"During the day and in the evening it is quite different".*

I began now to wash Margaret's hair for her. It was something that she agreed to readily and in truth I found that I enjoyed doing it for her. I actually became quite proficient at washing and blow drying her hair. She was blest with a head of black curls. She often used to say that she would have given anything to have had straight hair even though so many others would have given a lot to have hair like hers. It certainly was easy to maintain when short. It simply fell into place itself.

I took Margaret to her hairdresser regularly. She had been going to Mary's Hair Stylist shop at Stones Corner for many years. Mary always cut and coloured Margaret's hair for her personally. She was a most gentle and understanding woman who never made me or Margaret feel other than special customers. Margaret held Mary in the highest esteem.

There were many humorous incidents in our journey. I learned the hard way that if there was to be laughter then it had to be by mutual consent so that the sufferer did not feel in any way demeaned. So we did laugh when Margaret unbuckled her seat belt when we arrived home one day. She almost immediately forgot that she had done so and buckled herself up again. She could not understand why it was so difficult to exit the car.

Apart from a number of good books that I found in book stores, I would browse the internet to read as much as I could about Alzheimer's disease. In June one site I found seemed to suggest that most Alzheimer's disease contracted prior to age 60 is a familial type. That meant it was probably passed on to Margaret through her parents and she could have passed it on to one or more of our children. The rate of progression for the disease in such cases is much faster than the norm. That information made me sadder and naturally worried for our children's sake. It is a reason amongst others that I hope and pray for a cure before too many years have passed.

I used the internet to join a chat room on Alzheimer's. It was an American based chat room. In response to one of my questions I received a reply that suggested I was seeking answers in the wrong place. It was suggested that I correspond with a Dr Alan McCutcheon in Western Australia who, it was said, was a world expert. I did email him on several occasions and each time he responded very fully. His first reply I received on 23 June. He provided me with the clearest explanation of the disease and its implications that I had read to that time. He also suggested that I try the drug Aricept for Margaret, a matter I later took up with our neurologist.

We continued regular visits to our neurologist throughout the year. In preparation for our first visit on 18 January Margaret had her ceretec scan at the Mater. They had to take it twice as I recall. On the day of our visit Margaret was to have an EEG at 10.30am. We had an early morning storm which seemed to slow everyone down, but we made it just in time. Thankfully the doctor was himself a little late.

> *"The neurologist showed us the ceretex scan results and those of 12 months ago. Did the same with the EEG. They both show deterioration. While I have noted that, and I am sure Marg knows it too, it is of some pain to hear. He spoke of using Aricept. Even had some there. They cost $300 for 28 and have significant side effects. We decided not to use them at this time though. Again he says they are not a cure. Tells Marg just to hang in there, be active, read, exercise and enjoy life.*
> *We had a coffee and Marg was visibly upset. I feel so helpless and I am such a poor helper. I get short when she does silly things. I wish I were different. I told her again how much she is loved. We will not see her left without support. I just can't imagine how I would cope if the shoe were on the other foot. I too must re-evaluate my life and where my energies and priorities go."*

It strikes me now that we should have started the Aricept at this point. Its most likely effect would have been to have slowed the progression of the disease for a period of 6 to 18 months. However, nothing is gained by reflecting on what might have been for us. For other carers I do believe that to start as early as the doctor would suggest is worthwhile especially as there are some three or more drugs capable of slowing down the progression of the disease.

Later in the month I did approach our family doctor about the drug. He had a few elderly patients taking it. Only in one case did a patient react so violently that they had to come off it. As for all drugs, we would find by experience that each person may react differently to any one of them.

In April I again raised the issue of taking Aricept with our family doctor. The choice available for us was either to try Aricept or Exelon. Of the two, the side effects for Exelon were possibly more severe. Our doctor had been recently to a seminar outlining the most recent research on Alzheimer's and he thought that the use of one of the drugs and also vitamin E would be worth trying. He suggested that I would need to discuss this with the neurologist.

Margaret was due for her regular mammogram at QE 2 Hospital. In the past she had had a mild scare which later turned out not to be cancer. I was surprised how well she got through the ordeal. It was to be her last. From then on it was decided that she would not be able to manage the process. She had to sign a form in three places and did so quite comfortably. I filled out the rest of the form for her. It was interesting that even at this stage while she could sign her name she could not print it or simply write it. I suppose the act of signing was almost an automatic activity. The third of July finds this diary entry:

> *"The day we have grown to 'hate' was with us today. Marg and I met with the neurologist at 10.30. He was his usual 'cold' self; don't know how else he can be. He gave Marg tests – she could not remember his name, the day of the week, the year, etc. He got her to try to reproduce a drawing but she could not and was slow on some of the hand – eye stuff. Said he was sure Marg had Alzheimer's. I asked about Aricept. He had to contact Canberra about it, and then he has to do an EEG in a month. Told me there is nothing he can do for us and that we should begin to plan for the future. I was upset inside at his saying Marg had moderate to severe Alzheimer's. The speed of growth is throwing me. We did get the first lot of Aricept to take tonight. He warned us not to get up our hopes and if Marg got ill throw them away. I am so uptight about all this it is not funny. Marg too has been close to tears all day."*

Later that night I added:

> *"Can get angry with God, but to what effect. I just hope we do gain the graces needed for what life has ahead. Somehow we have to enjoy what life has to offer. There is much if we like to look at it positively."*

A month later Margaret and I returned to see the neurologist. She had her EEG even though it was now very difficult for her to remain still, not swallow, etc. We had come a week after our original appointment date as the doctor's father had died. Margaret was really sympathetic towards the doctor and it showed. She forgot her 'dislike' for him and became her normal self, showing feelings for the person and his loss. It was beautiful to see. After receiving the EEG results:

> "He showed us some signs that could lead to Margaret suffering epileptic fits. Her 'funny feeling' could be that. If they got worse or more frequent they can be controlled by tablets. Said that he thought Marg was more with it in his view. Aricept could be working."

This was a revelation to me as I reread my diary. In the busyness of my role as carer I lost sight of what he had to say that day with respect to possible epileptic fits. It pays to make notes of these things and refer to them occasionally during the progression of the disease.

Later in the year a new drug had come to my notice. It was called Reminyl. I was keen to try it, but first contacted Dr McCutcheon again. He warned me that if we were to change drugs and the drug did not work or was not accepted by the sufferer, then the sufferer would deteriorate and any loss in function would not be regained. I do believe it was his nice ways of saying to me, if Aricept is working don't change. That was 18 November. However, with our neurologist's blessing we did try Reminyl. The trial was a disaster. Within weeks all the family could see a major deterioration in Margaret, so we went back on to Aricept. My learning was that not everyone will react positively to new and 'better' treatments. Desperate people do desperate things though.

For the greater part of the year Margaret continued to assist with the washing and hanging out of the clothes. She would iron as long as I was there to assist and of course she loved our walks together. I would try to get her to take on other tasks:

> "Tried to get her to make a salad sandwich, but that was too much. She admitted to me that she finds it hard to find the correct page for the hymns at mass."

She would on occasion have little successes:

> "Marg stayed at home, but did set the table and I think was as proud of her effort as I was of her."

These successes were offset by what happened later the same day:

> "I was going to go to hit some golf balls. I thought I should check that Marg could ring me if needed. I was devastated to find she could not. She has little concept of numbers and just cannot dial the required numbers. I did not go out. I had her in tears. I just don't know how to help. Later we spent an hour trying to learn, but she could not. I did not realise how far this Alzheimer's has affected some of her functions."

I tried in the days ahead to buy a telephone on which I could preset the numbers. Margaret would simply have to press one number for each regular phone number. She could not choose the correct single number. At times like this I would feel the world closing around us and that we were trapped. I was seeing the world through my eyes without turning my full attention to how my dear wife must have been seeing the same world. A few days later:

> "We tried the phone again. I tried every which way to make it simple but Marg just got more and more confused. I try desperately to stay calm but cannot. I must frighten my poor struggling wife. I see the utter frustration in her. She feels so inadequate and I don't help. Even marked the phone with a marker pen, but that added to the confusion. Seems I need a phone or a pager with just one button to push. We gave up. It struck me that if I collapsed Marg could not get help for me by phone. That is scary."

To try to combat this we agreed that one of the girls would ring me each day to check that all was well. I soon learned that I had better answer the phone when it rang or I would receive several calls. I would receive the rounds of the table too if I did not take my mobile phone with me when away from home.

Margaret's ability to follow the simplest of instructions had deteriorated far more rapidly than I had expected. Early in November I note:

> "I asked her to open the nearest door on the kitchen cupboards. She says that she knows what a door is, but until I showed her she could not find the nearest. Instead she wanted to reach for things in a cupboard she had opened. It is all I can do not to cry. I cry internally and keep asking God why her. Surely if he could heal so many while he was on earth he could do so now for Marg. She has hurt no one. She is a beautiful person who loves God. We pray together most nights. We miss when I think she is too tired. Still I pray though poorly. I don't seem to be able to storm heaven. Perhaps I am lacking in true faith, perhaps I am not sure God will do it, that we are not important enough in the order of things."

At least by July, if not before then, I was fully aware that Margaret needed the level of support that was necessary for a very young child. She could no longer live alone and feed, clothe and fully care for her personal needs. I had to be constantly on guard to help her when and where she needed help. That tended to make me emotionally and physically very tired. For her part, Margaret told me that she was feeling depressed because she could no longer do what others could do. When she noticed I was feeling down she would wonder if I had the same problem as she did.

Early in September my dear wife shared with me that there were 'others' or 'people' in the house who were constantly moving and hiding her things. There were a myriad of little things that could be detailed about her behaviours from this time. I spent hours looking for her toothbrush as she loved to pick it up and carry it around the house with her and then 'lose' it. She would fold ever so neatly some of her clothes and then store them in her hiding places – behind the bedroom door, beside the dressing table, under cushions on the lounge chairs. She wanted to know how everyone else got fed since I was preparing tea for just the two of us. I never went out, other than to dash up to the corner store, without ensuring there was someone to stay with Margaret. Even so she told me in tears on 14 November that:

> "She did not want to be left alone."

I told her that would never happen. Earlier I wrote:

> "Marg had a bad night last night. At 2am I thought I should move out into a nearby room. Got some sleep but have a sore neck. At 6.15 went back to our bed. Poor Marg was in distress. She could not breathe well and she did not know where I had gone. She thought she had been left alone and did not know what to do. I could have cried - in fact I did secretly. She was so relieved to see me. She has a little incontinence at night - not every night - and that worried her too."

I mention incontinence twice in my diary for this year. It was not a major problem requiring intervention, but it did disturb Margaret when it occurred, usually towards morning. I had no idea the extent that incontinence would influence our lives in the years ahead. In hindsight I should have been more conscious about her drinking before bed at night. I should also have been aware how difficult it was becoming for Margaret to undo some of her clothing to attend to calls of nature. I have struggled within myself about mentioning anything at all with respect to incontinence in our journey with Alzheimer's. For the sufferer it is an undignified part of the realities of the disease. It is though part of the disease process, more so for some than for others. There is no blame. The sufferer's brain simply loses control over their ability to control bodily functions. To have excluded reference to incontinence and its effects on both of us would have been to falsify our story which I do not wish to do.

Though it is easy to write, as I have above, that there is no blame, I am ashamed to recall the times I laid blame. Again I have thought to leave such realities out of any recording of our journey. That too would be unfair and unrealistic. A carer will come to know their own humanity, their strengths and their weaknesses. I keep before me always the image of Jesus falling while carrying His cross and needing help along the way. I convinced myself that to fall was different to failing for as long as I could ask forgiveness, pull myself up and keep going. I would give everything never to have blamed Margaret for anything she did while suffering from this terrible disease, never to have been annoyed or angry. Perhaps in that case I would not have been human, certainly not the person I am.

In many respects I re-read my diaries with a great deal

of trepidation. Of their nature they are private musings in which I don't mind admitting my failings. So for 2001 at least I was pleased to note only 6 such references. In the first part of the year I was still struggling with the completion of consultancy work undertaken earlier, but I am honest enough to say:

> *"That is not an excuse for being short with Marg. I have to keep reminding myself that this is not a game. She genuinely cannot remember things. She is prone to taking 15 minutes to decide what to wear."*

And in February:

> *"I tried to get Marg to get her own cereal for breakfast. I think the exercise caused her to be embarrassed in front of her daughter. I, just for a change, got mad. Really I have no justification for that. If the shoe were on the other foot I would be utterly devastated. My prayer for me is that I may grow to be better at being a loving carer. I think my anger is more about my embarrassment that my highly intelligent wife now struggles with the simplest tasks. I am depressed with my own action and reaction."*

An entry I have for 20 August has an air of the comical about it. It is a pity that at the time I did not see that and have a laugh. My advice to carers is that they should look for the humorous in events and enjoy them for the relief they provide.

> *"My heart is heavy tonight because again I let myself get flustered at tea time and then got upset at Marg who was doing nothing. I had the tea on the go; the table had not been set, she needed nasal spray. I asked her to get it for me while I got something from the downstairs fridge. When I returned she had a pair of trousers I had worn earlier in the day out on the kitchen table. How could she confuse nasal spray with trousers? She may even be a little deaf of late. I cracked with the usual temper tantrum that goes with it. She looked horrified and cried. My heart sank. How dare I act so towards her in particular who for more than 33 years met my every need without complaint, and*

> *certainly without throwing a 'fit'. I apologised but that does not stop the hurt. She wants to help but needs simple one at a time instructions. I need God to walk with me, to help me serve her needs at this time."*

It may be important to acknowledge that at this point in the progression of the disease the sufferer does desperately want to feel helpful and useful. Similarly it is important to understand that what the carer sees as a simple task is rather complex for the sufferer. When a direction is given, the carer should be open to its being carried out in a way the carer may find hard to imagine. This is the nature of the life now shared. There is humour, and laughter has a healing effect. Yet the carer has to contend with the daily grind. The carer seldom gets a break from all the little problems not yet seen by others. It really is difficult to accept what is happening to the one so loved. I reflected on 20 November:

> *"I must internally come to grips with the fading memory and severe loss of language and then treat her with the love and care she deserves. I am chastened when I think of how she would care for me if the circumstances were reversed."*

The carer's ability to accept what happens daily will, in my experience, be tested by the sufferer offering excuses and even being in total denial of what they have obviously done. It is much like the action of the young child. With Margaret I feel sure it was a mixture of simply forgetting that she had done things coupled with the fear of her seeing me annoyed at her.

My final thoughts about the year 2001 are the hardest to relate. The impact at the time hurt me very deeply and maybe for that reason I had almost put the event out of my mind. It has been rather difficult to revisit this part of our journey, but I am sure it is one other carers will also have to face. I will let my diary entry of 19 May speak for itself:

> *"Marg last night said she did not know we were married. Had trouble with the concept of me as husband though she knows she loves me. Found that very hard to take. Have to keep reminding myself that her memory is being eroded. Perhaps I*

had hoped it would not get to this. Lord help her. Lord help me to understand, accept what can't be changed and to always be able to help Marg. I dread the future."

In a couple of weeks after that event, we went walking in Fehlberg Park. Margaret wanted a swing so I gave her one. As we walked:

"She held my hand and told me she was so pleased I was with her."

Then two days later after she had had her afternoon rest:

"She tells me she really loves me when I am happy. I should be more careful to be happy about her. I do get tired at times. All part of the carer's learning curve."

And again on 5 July:

"She asked me tonight what I was doing here and how I got here. I think she was wanting to know how we met and married. I went through our story with her. She tells me she loves me and does not want to lose me."

On 5 August we attended a party put on for Margaret's youngest brother. He was turning 50. Margaret enjoyed the experience and I noted:

"One great outcome was that she finally figured where I fitted in. I think I look so different in our wedding pictures she wondered how I got involved. She is so pleased to understand. I could cry but know that things are likely to get worse."

Sadly by the night of 5 September my dearest Margaret:

"Did not know my name, did not know I was her husband. I was 'a nice man.'"

I suppose it was then only a matter of time before Margaret would get to the point I outline on 24 September:

> "I am still getting over an event of this morning. I am going to have to get used to these things, but it is hard. Marg had been ironing. She came out to the kitchen and I sensed she was upset. I asked what was up. She had tears in her eyes as she told me she wanted to go home. She missed her family and wanted to be with them. I asked where home was and she told me where her mother was. I fought against the hurt welling up inside of me and talked about our home. Told her she was a mother and we had lived in this home for longer than she had ever spent at 'home'. Eventually said she understood but I don't think she does understand 'marriage' or 'husband' etc. I thought she may grow a little better, but I don't think that is the case. Even late today I am cut up inside but guess others go through this."

This theme of going home increased over time as the disease deepened. Eventually I grew to accept it as part of the disease's progression, but there was always some pain in doing so.

> "I can sense losing her as I know her. I have tried to tell myself that she has to be the centre of my life even if/when I am not that for her. I feel very lonely at times and scared of what the future holds for us both. I am not made for this. God certainly hands out the challenges."

I thought towards the end of the year, 26 November, that it may be helpful to go through our wedding album together. It was after all her prized possession which she kept in a drawer away for the kids as they were growing up.

> "Marg got quite distressed when we went through our wedding album. She has no recollection of that day. Feels it has been kept from her. She was quite distressed really. I was surprised. It is such a shame. This disease is a monster. She is not even aware that she has a disease now I think."

The tone for the year is captured in my entry for Christmas Day:

> "My heart is heavy as I write. I am not sure where my lovely wife is in her head. She is not happy. Does not know where she

should be. I sense she feels she should be with her family i.e. brothers and sisters, not her own children. I can never be sure who she thinks I am. She looks so lost and I feel powerless to fill the void."

Still the carer has to fill the void. I now also believe that the carer needs a confidant to whom he/she can download the emotional issues faced and seek balance so as to be better able to carry out such a demanding role. To an extent I found my confidant in my parish priest, Brendan. However the level of demand would, like most other things in life, be revealed only in stages.

Chapter 5

2002

An Adult as Child

*T*welve months in our journey with early onset Alzheimer's is a very long time. Changes come thick and fast and from the carer's point of view you hardly have time to adjust to one change when another is upon you. Your powers to adapt are stretched to the limit, at least mine were. That is enough though about the mythical 'you' as carer. This story is about Margaret's and my journey in which, as carer, I had to learn to cope with both success and failure. However I do pray that every carer will be given the strength necessary to carry out what each one is called upon to do.

This year I would gain a deep appreciation for how a person is affected by sleep deprivation. I found it was extremely difficult for me to control my mood swings so as to remain calm in all circumstances. Calmness in the face of the daily grind is what the sufferer looks for, indeed I think expects. From the start of the year I was called upon to do everything – washing, ironing, cooking, shopping, cleaning, bathing, and so the list goes on. On top of finding time to do all the necessary daily chores, I had to be sure to take care of the personal needs of the most precious gift in my life – my Margaret.

For me the most difficult aspect of caring was dealing with incontinence. Perhaps if I had some background in nursing or other medical occupation I would not have found it so foreign a matter to cope with. In late 2001 Margaret did have some loss of normal bladder control especially at night. I thought I had that relatively under control through the use of incontinence pads. Thank God I had three daughters to advise me here. I soon became a fair expert on the type of pads available, their strengths and weaknesses. I even lost my embarrassment standing in front of those rows of pads at the supermarket and sussing out what was best, let alone going through the checkout with them. I did have trouble on occasion convincing Margaret to wear one each night, especially as they needed to be more bulky. As time went by one of the little 'games' we would have was 'find the pad'. If Margaret decided to discard one during the night while I was asleep, she was never able to remember where she placed it.

Faecal incontinence is another level altogether. I used to find it relatively easy to change the nappies of my own children when they were little, and now can force myself to do the same for my grandchildren in an emergency. I did not believe that I could ever do the same for an adult. I am here to say it is surprising what you can do for another whom you love and who is in desperate need of your help.

I do regret having to write about this part of our journey because I in no way want to sully the memory of my beautiful wife. It is, however, as I have said elsewhere, a part of our journey's reality and to pretend it is not would be to lie. I may though be forgiven for leaving out details not necessary to follow our journey.

On Sunday, 13 January, we rose early to get ready to attend mass. I found Margaret in the bathroom highly distressed. She had had a bowel movement. The toilet in our home is situated some distance from the bathroom. In the months ahead I learned that sometimes she simply could not find the toilet. Putting up signs was of little use as she could not read signs all that well. I wondered this day how I would cope, yet I did. I showered her, cleaned up, washed the soiled clothes and wrote:

"I hope that was a one off."

Bed wetting was now largely under control with the use of the bulkier pads. I found that 'Tina' or 'Depend' worked adequately and were tolerated well by Margaret. As to my reaction to having sometimes to change bedclothes and her pyjamas during the night, I write on 25 March:

> "I regret that I treat her like a naughty child, then I look after her. How poor is that! She tries so hard to be normal. I hope God can forgive me and give me the graces I need now and in the future."

We began to have a problem with faecal incontinence after our daily walk. I also found that with the door of the toilet closed when not in use, Margaret would assume it was in use. She would then look for another place to use. Some time later I determined to leave the door always open with a light on day and night. Still:

> "I get so cross because I can't understand this to be my Margaret. I settle knowing it is not the woman even of 12 months ago. I do find it so hard to cope though."

When soiling was an issue, Margaret's own reaction was interesting. After a 3am incident on 2 April:

> "Poor darling was ashen, shaking and highly embarrassed though putting the blame on the other lady."

It was no doubt her way of coping. Reminded me of the child who says it was not me. I only wish I could have thought along such lines at the time.

I was now supervising Margaret's daily shower. She would allow me to help, but with some reluctance. Towelling herself was her job totally. While she had always preferred a hot bath rather than a shower, she found getting into and out of the tub just too difficult even with my assistance. There was always the chance of her slipping. As the incidences of incontinence grew, I invested in a hand held shower. Later again I purchased one where the control of water flow was located at the head of the shower rose. That was an invaluable investment which saved me showering myself every time I had to let go of the shower to assist in other ways.

As I assume one does with a child, I would always try to get Margaret to use the toilet before we went out. I grew to know the body language of need as, I notice, mothers do. Even so on 9 June:

> *"Marg got toey and we crossed swords because she got cross at me for asking if she wanted to use the toilet. I can tell often when she needs to."*

Such events kept reminding me that I was caring for an adult whose brain was affected by a disease making it virtually impossible for her to act as she had acted all her adult life. There is a fine line to be walked by the carer throughout this stage because there are many lucid moments. I experienced this after Margaret thought the bathroom was the toilet in early July:

> *"She told me perhaps she should go away. I told her she will be with me and I would care for her."*

As I look back on 2002, I realise that some of my frustration and Margaret's embarrassment could have been avoided by better supervision. I am sure, for example, that having reached the toilet during the night, Margaret could just not remember what next to do. She may not have accepted my help in such a private activity, but perhaps I should have been more forceful in offering to help. I will never know now, though it is worth thinking about for others.

By October I was getting up 2 to 3 times a night to ensure Margaret reached the toilet. I had erected a sensor light on the way from our bedroom to the toilet to ensure Margaret had a lighted passage at least. It was not as successful as I had hoped. There were too many ways one could take to reach the toilet. We were still sleeping together in our queen sized bed. I was thus generally aware when Margaret would stir and be on the move.

Incontinence certainly places a strain on the carer to be ever watchful and alert or pay the consequences. In early November:

> "After breakfast I suggested that Marg go to the toilet. I could hear her moving around and should have known that she could not find the toilet. Having so much loose furniture on the verandah threw her. I get annoyed as I should not do. With tears in her eyes she told me she was really trying. I am still crying to myself as I have done several times today when I remember the scene."

How devastating must it have been for Margaret to realise that she could no longer even control fully her normal bodily functions no matter how much she tried. There was no way she could overcome the lack of control. Imagine too the pain she must have felt when her carer would at times go off his brain at her. I recall this particularly when she had a bout of diarrhoea. That led to another issue for me – how to treat a raw and burned behind. Once more my daughters and their mothering skills came to the rescue. I found myself getting to know about the various barrier creams and water repellents from the baby section of the supermarket shelves.

Unfortunately for us both, incontinence was to be a 'normal' part of our daily existence from this point onwards. Losing my temper about it accomplished nothing in the long run other than to be an outlet for my frustrations. Whenever I stayed calm and fully supportive, Margaret reacted with such gentleness in return.

I thought that I was having a bad time of it in 2002. Little did I realise what lay ahead in the years to follow. I noted that I recorded 50 incontinence incidents during 2002, and that meant that the other 300 or so days were clear. Later those numbers would change dramatically.

Our daily life was not always troublesome, though it was seldom easy. Even when we took little journeys and holidays we had our moments of concern, but they were mainly times of joy. In fact I gained the impression on a number of occasions that Margaret did not want to return home. The breaks were good for the two of us. It was our way of trying to make the best of the hand we had been dealt.

In early January we, Margaret with our youngest daughter Anne and me, journeyed first to Sydney and then to Melbourne.

I would never have attempted such holidays without having another person with me. To have a woman to assist Margaret in public in particular was essential, although I do believe that Anne's presence was meeting my security need rather than Margaret's. It was to be expected that, when away from home, Margaret would experience some level of confusion. The confusion grew worse when we had to ask for a new room soon after settling in because the toilet was leaking.

> "Marg has been a handful. I think she is really confused, misses home and its secure environment. Wonders what she can do. I almost cry as I help her bath, dress, etc. Even in eating she is confused and walked away with one of the napkins."

I learned early on in our journey with Alzheimer's that, if a decision is made to have a holiday that decision should be made after considering all the possible eventualities. For example in our case Margaret's normal day involved her spending a lot of time in her bedroom. I was also aware that she did not like eating out when she thought people were staring at her. Knowing these things helped me prepare for some disruptions. I was pleasantly surprised how well Margaret coped with plane travel and most other aspects of the travel itself. The bonus was having Anne with us. I have often wondered how much of a genuine holiday it was for her. Our girls are the great legacy Margaret has left me.

When we ate out the food served for Margaret had to be simple fare and easy to eat. She was too embarrassed to try anything out of the ordinary. She also had a fear of being left alone while we were sight seeing. I needed to hold her hand and be sure to have her comfort seen to at all times. Once she felt safe and secure she was happy. It again brought home to me how important was the security she now felt in her own home.

While at Melbourne we took the Great Southern Coast Road tour. It began early in the morning and it was 10.30pm by the time we got back to our hotel. During the tour I had another major learning:

> "Marg gets disoriented at toilets. Thank God for Anne. I really don't know if we can travel alone anymore. She got stressed

on the way home. Just too long a journey for one day. Says she
enjoyed it though. Love her and can't understand why God the
Father in His compassion allows this to her."

Our next holiday involved going to the north coast on 21
May. Our middle daughter, Megan, was holidaying there with
her husband Ben. Margaret was once more confused and anxious
about her new environment. We had a great view of the ocean
which she loved and she indicated that she was looking forward
to walking along the beach. It was there that I had a beautiful
incident which I will forever treasure.

> "After breakfast we went for a walk to the beach. I tried to get
> Marg to put her feet in the water. Failed. When we sat on the
> sand together she actually lent over and gave me a kiss. First
> for months. It made my day."

About a month after we had returned home Megan called
in on 7 June.

> "Told me it was an eye opener up the coast to be with Marg
> and see what a fulltime job it is to look after her. She offers to
> give me a day off if I want it. I really appreciate the offer and no
> doubt will need help in the future."

Towards the end of June we travelled with our close
friends – Cath, Marcel, Ian and Gail - to Stanthorpe. We thought
it might be good for us to experience some really cold weather,
log fires and visit some wineries. Margaret enjoyed the drive,
especially the stop at Warwick to have lunch and to shop a
little. Cath and Gail always wanted to shop. We were joined at
Stanthorpe by Joe and Judy to complete the foursome of couples.
The few days at Stanthorpe were good though Margaret hated
the cold. Our return journey did have its moments.

> "We stopped at Warwick for a sandwich and drink. Marg got
> funny after that. Had to lock the car doors as I could not get her
> to understand we were on the way home."

Thank God that was the only time this type of thing happened. Margaret kept trying to take off her seatbelt and open the door of the car while we were driving. It was afternoon and I began to realise how insecure Margaret became when not indoors, in her secure place, as the sun begins to set.

Our final break away from home for the year was in December. This time we went to Noosa. Here we spent our honeymoon in 1965 at Bailey's Motel. How things had changed, both for Noosa and for us. On the day we set out for our holiday my poor girl had a bout of diarrhoea. Her bottom was sore from an incident a day earlier and this just exacerbated the problem for her. On Anne's suggestion I gave Margaret some Lomotil to control the diarrhoea and it eventually did the trick. Our eldest daughter, Maree, with her husband Michael and their two children Emer and Thomas were with us. It was a time largely of great joy. Our wedding anniversary falls on 11 December. It was good to celebrate this with those we loved so much. I wrote that night:

> *"37 years Marg and I have been married. For 34 years of that it has been truly magnificent. I thank God for bringing us together, for the beautiful people we have helped create and form, for our own love and respect for one another. There is so much to be thankful for it is hard to pit it against the sadness of our recent life together. I am not sure how much Marg recognised about the significance of today. I am filled with the thought that she relies on me like Maree's children rely on her. Yet she holds me in her hands while I kneel beside her and we pray our Pater Noster, three Hail Mary's and a Glory Be each night. Lord only knows what is in store for us, but I know we need God with us to succeed."*

Throughout the year we continued our regular walking and reading. In time the latter became more my reading to Margaret than her trying to read at all. Even by February I note:

> *"Marg and I went for a walk around the block after dropping off the car. Later I got her to read a little. She is much less able than a few months ago. I then read to her. She seems to enjoy that."*

What she really did enjoy was our sitting in the lounge room singing hymns. She would try to join in with those she could recall and at other times just hum along with me. I enjoyed that time also.

Any visit to our daughters was usually a time of joy. Margaret loved her little granddaughter, Emer, very much. Nevertheless I had to be careful not to overstay our visits. In the latter part of the year in particular, Margaret grew anxious after visiting for an hour or so. The only way to deal with this was for us to return home. The family accepted it as normal, but the wider community we moved within found it a little more difficult to understand.

Early on in the year I would learn that there were some no go areas as far as Margaret was concerned. On 18 January we were visiting friends, Brian and Margaret. I simply asked at one point if we had informed them about Margaret's Alzheimer's. That acted as a trigger.

> *"Marg reacted heatedly – wanted to know what was wrong with her, said I really don't like her and got up and stormed out saying she was going home and did not want to see me again. I apologised then caught up to her near the park. Says she knew where she was going. Got her home and put her to bed in a very distressed state. I am shattered too."*

Never in our 37 years of marriage had I witnessed Margaret so act. It was totally contrary to her nature. I would endeavour never to again discuss her condition with others in her presence. By the next day she was very much aware that she had insulted our friends. That was typical of my Margaret. Though they never believed it necessary:

> *"She suggested we go to see them soon to patch things up."*

Although Margaret could no longer remember how to operate the washing machine, she did continue to help me. She would arrange the clothes to go on the line and try to peg out some of the smaller items. As to the ironing, I record on 13 June:

> *"Later there was the washing to bring in and some ironing. Marg announced out of the blue that she is not going to iron anymore."*

Another job was thus added to the list for the carer. I secretly admired her courage to so opt out. I have no idea why she did other than she was finding it difficult to figure out how to iron the shirts, and I believe she may have been scared of the heat of the iron. I note in March for example that she had tried to iron without turning it on. Only after I turned it on and ironed a handkerchief did she seem to recall how to go ahead. Margaret however always wanted to help, often in ways that were a hindrance. She needed things to occupy her.

> *"I did the ironing in the morning. It was building up again. Marg has the idea that she needs to fold things. She took a couple of shirts I had ironed, folded them and put them in the drawer. Why iron."*

The only time Margaret had ever folded my shirts was when she was packing a suitcase for me. These types of behaviours were part and parcel of our journey throughout 2002. The carer would do well to be able to see the humour in such cases.

Attending mass of a weekend was always an integral part of our religious observance. It was my aim to have us attend mass together for as long as possible. I knew that Margaret would want that. If it was my turn to be the Reader or Eucharistic minister, I worried that Margaret might try to come up from the congregation to the altar to be with me. I think the fact that I could always be seen by her from the body of the church was sufficient security for her.

Margaret loved the singing of hymns. If there was a choir to belong to she would always want to be part of it. Now my dear wife could not even find the right page of the hymnal. Rather than embarrass her by having to find the correct page for her, we began to sing off the one book. Not everything went smoothly while attending mass. On 13 April:

> *"We went to mass. Marg for the first time carried the host back to her seat and I had to tell her to eat it. She was upset after when I told her of that. She says to me, when I am frustrated at her not being able to do simple things, 'Vince I am really trying hard'. I feel such a bastard. I am sure God tut-tuts at me as well."*

Attempts to ensure that Margaret could use her signature if required became very difficult. When she would practice for me, the first attempt would be good, but after that it would deteriorate rapidly. By April Margaret even found it difficult to write out the letters of the alphabet. She no longer wanted to practise writing. I noted also that she now had little time for her reading glasses. Though she had worn them for the better part of her life, she discarded them completely. I guess she did not read anymore and she could see well enough for ordinary purposes without them. It meant too that there was one less thing for her to remember.

Margaret's short term memory was waning noticeably. We had been out all morning on 19 April with our daughter, Maree, and our granddaughter, Emer.

> *"After lunch at home I told Marg what we had done in the morning. She was in tears because she wanted to see Emer and Maree and I could not convince her she had been there with me."*

Margaret returned to taking Aricept after the failure of the Reminyl tablets trialled at the end of 2001. She certainly appeared much more her 'old self' once they got into her system. Unfortunately this drug also had a limited term of effectiveness. It could only slow the progression somewhat, not cure. When Margaret would regress it was obvious, hence my comment on 6 May:

> *"Marg seems to be having one of those days where she appears to have moved down the scale. She is quiet and somewhat removed."*

At such times the rate of change would often be significant:

> *"It actually gets harder each day to keep up with the changes in Marg. She finds it hard to sit still, her conversation is muddled, she confuses me with someone else, she is having more trouble swallowing tablets, etc."*

A few days after that reflection, I took Margaret to have her hair done - cut and colour - at Stones Corner. She looked very smart afterwards. Later that day though:

> "Mary rang me in the afternoon to say Marg had put on a turn. Did not want to stay. Thought it was taking too long. Wanted to wait outside, etc. Mary was most sympathetic. I apologised and said I would sit around in the salon next time. Marg has been agitated all day."

At her next appointment on 18 July I stayed with Margaret. Over time I became part of the furniture so to speak. I found I needed to take a book with me as the women's magazines were just not my cup of tea. I did once or twice have my eyebrows clipped for free. Mary, Margaret's hairdresser and the owner, commented on how much more relaxed Margaret was with my being present.

By 18 June I was finding that Margaret's ever declining language skills were a problem for us both.

> "Marg and I are getting off on the wrong foot often. It is usually over nothing and often I am not aware what the problem is. Marg's language skill has so declined I can't often tell what she is trying to say is the problem. She uses words, but the words do not make a coherent sentence. That frustrates her as well."

Towards the end of the year, 1 November to be exact, my darling had developed a head cold. This would again show me how dependent she now was fast becoming. She would at times have great difficulty trying to blow her nose. It hurts somewhat to have to try to teach your adult wife how to do what appears to be so simple an action. In time, of course, she would not be able to independently carry out even this basic action. Other problems followed this as I wrote on 6 December:

> "Having a problem more and more of getting Marg to eat meals. She seems to eat half a sandwich for example, then lose interest. She may rearrange her food on her plate but does not eat. I can't talk to her about it. It just adds to my frustration. Guess she won't let herself starve."

In the light of the future for my Margaret I realise how ironic that final remark of mine was. By 18 December another area of change was evident:

> "Marg seems to have found a new friend. She is spending a lot of time in front of the mirror – door to the clothes cupboard in Maree's old room. She seems to talk to her own image. I suggested to her it was herself. She scoots out of the room now when she sees me coming."

Once again my judgement was clouded to say the least. I was embarrassed by seeing my highly intelligent Margaret in conversation with her own image. They would even touch one another. I was always cleaning the hand marks off the mirror. That Margaret did not recognise her own image was too hard for me to accept. I should have realised that the disease had so affected her mind that she now remembered herself as a much younger person than that portrayed in her mirror image. One of the most endearing images of this turn of events happened a few days later on the day before Christmas.

> "I had a little cry to myself this morning. As we came upstairs Marg saw her image in the mirror doors in Maree's old room. She beamed and rushed to say hello to her image and to introduce me. I have tried telling her she is talking to herself. Note she spends a lot of time there. She tries to touch the image – the glass is always dirty after I clean it. Tonight she told me of this nice girl, about her age, quite young Marg thought, how polite she is to talk to. Can this be any worse than talking to dolls? She talks to and touches images of the grandchildren on the computer screen."

In her newly developing world she had a friend. I soon accepted the image as her friend because that friend would turn up in the most unexpected places, namely everywhere there was a mirror. I was embarrassed early on in shopping centres and the like, but eventually I even felt comfortable there too. After all my beautiful wife had thought well enough of me to have formally introduced us on 24 December.

During 2002 Margaret continued to have her episodes or 'turns'. As early as 28 February I record:

> "Marg woke feeling unwell. She looked pale and got cold and clammy. She spent most of the day lying down and did not eat well."

When next it occurred it was in the morning, but it was her headache that caused most concern. Sleep seemed to be the only cure. Then there was a change on 6 April:

> "We had a strange occurrence during the early morning. It was about 5am when Marg woke me with her cries. She was asleep, but obviously having a nightmare. She was terrified, but could not tell me what it was about. It took 12 minutes or so for her to calm down. Half an hour later she was at it again."

A few days later she told me that something funny had happened in her head. The next morning:

> "Marg had a little head turn again today. She tells me there is no pain. She then tells me a story. It must be that she experiences a jumble of thoughts or visions."

Following this Margaret would tell me of other people who were in the house although we were definitely alone. I suppose it could simply have been her own image that she noticed as she passed by the many mirrors in the house. Hallucinating accompanies this disease. There was certainly another change in behaviour, one that would worsen as the years went by. It involved the change in her demeanour in the afternoons. I believe this is often referred to as the 'sundowners' syndrome. On 2 February:

> "I note that after a rest in the afternoon Marg invariably looks agitated. Tells me she is wondering how she will get home. Needs to check on her family. I don't think that means her own children. I try to tell her this is her home, but that does little to allay her fears. I then try to get her involved with me in some activity."

At times there was a little humour in the situations that evolved. I always had to ensure that if I were to laugh it had to be done in such a way that Margaret did not think it was directed at her. She had had her afternoon nap one day and then:

> "Kept telling me of a man sitting on the front verandah. I asked her where? It was me she was thinking of - at lunch time."

We normally sat on the verandah to eat our lunch together and watch TV. It was not easy to know what to say, how to say it, or when to say it at this point in the disease's progression.

To feel secure of an evening was paramount in Margaret's life needs. A little snippet from 25 May does, I hope, illustrate the point.

> *"One run in with Marg in the evening. We had been over to Anne's for tea. Marg seemed tense about it all and wanted to come home. We left after washing up. I told Marg that that was not nice and she denied she wanted to come home. Got upset that I was upset with her. I get lost at times trying to figure out what to do, when to be quiet."*

Of an afternoon I sometimes wondered whether Margaret would wander away from home. Once in a while she would go to the front door, but could not figure out how to open the security door. A short walk was normally all that was required for her to settle down.

We had several meetings with our neurologist throughout the year. The first meeting was on 5 February. Her fear of these visits was premised on her hatred of

> *"Being made a 'fool' of as she puts it."*

The usual testing of her word skill indicated how much it had declined in a short period. He believed, as did I, that the Aricept was helping to give Margaret a better quality of life. He said that we all react differently to various drugs so that it did not concern him that the Reminyl had not worked for her.

On May 23 it was to be me who had a mild panic attack. Margaret had pointed out to me that there was blood on her pad. I changed the pad and after we had been for our morning walk there was another show. I almost lost it. I had all sorts of thoughts and to add to my distress was the fact that our family doctor was on vacation. I contacted Margaret's mother who advised that I should have it checked out as soon as possible.

I now had to do something that I assume a carer never thinks they will have to do, particularly if the carer is male. Thinking that she may have a bladder infection, I needed to have a urine sample to take with me. Somehow I was successful in doing so. I explained Margaret's condition to the doctor. We had at various times over 30 or so years been to all three doctors in the surgery. The doctor who saw Margaret was so gentle and nice with her. Thankfully there was no bladder infection. With the nurse's assistance the doctor was successful in obtaining a cervical scrape for testing and ordered an ultrasound for the following day.

> "She handled it very well but is confused about it all. Got depressed. Said she may not see us all much longer – I cried yet again."

I expected the next day to be very trying.

> "I could sense Marg was anxious though she conducted herself beautifully throughout the ordeal. I could not get her to drink the one and a half litres of water required before we left home at 9am. As a result they had to do an internal scan. They wondered how Marg would cope, but she was fine."

Our doctor later informed us that there were no abnormalities. He would review this when he had the results of the pap smear test.

It was 5 August when we next visited the neurologist. I remember that it turned out to be a very emotionally draining day for us both. Even after 6 months Margaret hated to go. Her distress was always based on her fear of being tested only to 'fail' each time. When he had completed his battery of tests, the doctor:

> "Said her language had been shot, that she also has trouble doing hand movements, etc. None of this is news to me but I don't want it confirmed. He said he would see us in 6 months as long as coming was not a stress on Margaret. Told me to plan now for her to be institutionalised. I hate that. Has been on my mind all day and Marg caught me crying as I was looking at her in the afternoon. Dr says she is a lucky woman to have someone like me looking after her and her family's support. Told me to look after myself too. Marg got annoyed. Often picks up on what is said though can't express it."

It would be another three years before Margaret would enter a nursing home. Notwithstanding the doctor's counsel, what I did not do well was look after myself. In truth, the carer cannot function to the full extent if he/she does not take time out regularly to recharge the batteries, and does so without a feeling of guilt accompanying that R&R. If I had my time again, I would give myself more quality time out because, I now realise, the level of my caring would benefit, thus creating a better environment for the person being cared for by me.

I wonder today how I ever got through the years with the amount of broken sleep that is part of the lot of the carer. I felt this lack of sleep throughout 2002, but that was only a foretaste of what lay ahead. We were still sleeping in the one bed as I mentioned earlier. Perhaps it would have been wiser to have moved to single beds sooner than in fact we did. I am sure that I kept putting that move off because I sensed that Margaret would get very anxious if she woke and found I was not close by her. So our sleep was broken every night at least once for Margaret to visit the toilet. More disturbing was her newly developed ability to snore loudly and often. She loved to sleep on her back. I could normally get her to roll over, but there were times I figured it was best for her not to be disturbed and for me just to retire to one of our nearby bedrooms. On 27 September:

> "We had a terrible night last night. Marg would not roll off her back so at 1.30am I went into the next bedroom. I did not sleep well though. At 3.30 I was awoken by her crying out in terror. She has a nightmare on occasion. She would not go back to sleep after that and was up walking around by 6.30."

Margaret would wake with the dawn. Closing the blinds had little effect. Once awake she would lie in bed playing with her fingers and no matter how tired I was I would feel the movement. Sleeping in was not an option. Margaret, by the way, had always been one to go to bed early and sleep in when possible. I was always a person who went to bed late and was a fairly early riser. Now she would at least stay up until about 10pm.

Our time together after the evening meal was the most peaceful of the day. We would sit and watch TV together, not that Margaret followed much of what was going on. I believed she liked being beside me with no distractions, feeling safe and secure after her bath and tea. Sleep deprivation had its effect on Margaret also. In her case I was usually able to convince her to rest or have a short nap after lunch.

> "Marg had a good lunch and I talked her into having a good sleep. She seemed more like her 'usual' self after the sleep. Just wonder whether too little sleep affects her."

There are a few passages in my diary for 2002 that highlight the effect of sleep deprivation on me as carer. I cannot stress enough how important it is for the carer to try to have sufficient sleep. I am sure now that my impatience, indeed anger, was exacerbated by allowing myself to become overtired, by believing I did not need help, that I was invincible. It was Margaret's quality of life that would be adversely affected by my not reaching out for the help available to me. I write on 2 July:

> "Come the end of each day of late I am ready to leave - not that I would - but I am emotionally and physically drained. I have myself to look after as well as Marg full-time. She has mood swings and I am sure she gets bored from doing next to nothing. She breathes heavily often and mumbles to herself. Our 'conversations' have less and less meaning. It feels at times as though I am in a prison."

I now had a constant knot in my gut. Much of my day was spent in trying to be aware of Margaret's mood swings and then interpreting what they may mean for both of us. Towards the end of the year it was common for me to record:

> "Very tired during the day. Just had an overwhelming desire to close my eyes and sleep."

Life does go on no matter how differently. I figured that we should take whatever opportunities presented for us to be with friends. By now we had very few really good friends, people who could be with Margaret in public, support her and show no sense of embarrassment. Such people are worth their weight in gold at any time in life, but especially so for us at that time. For her part Margaret sensed their being non-judgemental and enjoyed their company. She felt safe and loved. Our outings were essential for me also as they helped to bring some sense of normalcy back into play. So in January we had a day at the races and dinner at Breakfast Creek afterwards. Margaret enjoyed going to the races though we did not often go. She was tired out after dinner so we returned home leaving the others to soldier on for a few more hours.

All outings were times that could prove difficult. We had a morning in town shopping and then stopped at the Shingle Inn for a cuppa with Megan.

> *"Noted that Margaret gets tired on these outings – could be the crowds. Loud noise agitates her."*

Loud noise was certainly a problem. It grew to the point where Margaret would even walk away from family celebrations when noise levels grew. Strangely though, we went to see a musical, "Singing in the Rain", and Margaret thoroughly enjoyed it. Music was a passion of hers.

We attended two birthday parties. As long as Margaret felt acknowledged she was fine. At one event Joe demanded that we all had to have something to say. I was so pleased that there was no thought of leaving Margaret out of this activity.

> *"Marg spoke well. She said it was great to be with people you know and like."*

At a larger party though I would record:

> *"Love to see Marg's face light up when she sees those whom she loves. Gets distressed when some do not know how to interact with her."*

I believe this is my first reference to a response that became her signature when this terrible disease took from Margaret her ability to speak coherently. I refer to her beaming smile of recognition. It would speak volumes.

It may be difficult at any time to gauge the level of frustration felt by either the carer or the sufferer, but frustration there is. How each one deals with it makes a difference. In saying that, I have no idea how my beautiful wife could have acted in any other way than the way she did in all circumstances. Imagine her frustration in thinking that our children were still living with us although they had left home long ago. I tried to capture some of that in my diary note of 16 February:

> *"I have one distressed and very confused wife today. It has been bad, yet good. She seems tired. She wanted to go somewhere at tea time. I could not understand where. She is anxious not to hurt me she says, but seems not to understand that the kids have left home. She wants them around and is fed up with doing nothing. I run out of ideas. Find it hard to get done what needs to be done and have a constant itinerary for her."*

Her boredom would often come through. Only after she found her 'friend' in the mirror did she become more accepting of her lot. As for myself, my frustrations would filter to the surface with greater strength and regularity as time and the disease marched on. I wrote about it on 3 March:

> *"Boy I am in one shit of a mood tonight. I am not sure why. I know I feel tired, I know sometimes I could scream at Marg's stupidity and I know this reaction is one I have chosen. None of those is to blame, though I want to blame. The girls have been around today. Marg wants them but finds it hard to place who they are. I can see she gets distressed when I am in a mood. She should not have to bear that on top of everything. I love family around, I can't imagine life without them, yet I get tired. I seem to have more to do. I am finding it hard to speak with Jesus, yet I speak. I ask for Marg's cure and see the opposite. I listen to hear God's voice, yet there is only deafening silence. My faith needs only to be as a mustard seed, mine must be so much smaller than that. I am not the stuff martyrs and saints are made of. I am weak though appearing strong. God, at least be my strength."*

People would often comment to me how well I was doing. They marvelled at how well I appeared to cope with all that was demanded of me. Little did they know of the inner turmoil. I can't imagine any carer not going through the same or similar inner conflict whether they overtly admit to it or not. My diary of 27 July again expresses some of my frustration.

> *"I risk repeating myself, but some days I want to scream. I get so frustrated that this wonderfully intelligent woman I have called my wife for 36 years is now so much a little child going backwards. She does not recognise me all the time, she will spend most of her day in our bedroom at the dresser, she will repeat, 'Um Hum' over and over. Still she relies so much on me and in her own way I am sure she loves me. I ask God to heal her, but the silence is deafening. I find excuses for God's seeming inactivity, even my words here are an excuse. I am tired of not being able to put my needs first, of having to come after. What a learning for me."*

Frustration was always a two way street. I got frustrated and annoyed because I could not understand what Margaret was trying to relate to me. She surely must have been even more frustrated at not being able to express her thoughts. Imagine also how it must be to find that in the afternoon you had very little recall of the events of that morning, let alone of the week just passed.

> *"Marg was in tears at breakfast. I gathered it was because she feels her mother never comes to see her. I can never get her to understand that we see Bernie regularly – twice this week. Later in the day she was crying to herself also, but I do not know why."*

It was November when other daily functions became difficult. Margaret actually came to tell me that she had no idea how to clean her teeth. For a time I found that if I showed her the action she could then manage. Taking large tablets was a problem. She always did have trouble swallowing them. Now she became very adept at hiding them behind her teeth. I could give her a glass of water which she would drink and that left me thinking the tablets were swallowed. I would often find these tablets later on the sink or in one of her regular hiding places. When the tablets were for her blood pressure the effect could be interesting to say the least.

I liked to take Margaret out as often as possible, but eating while out was becoming stressful for her. On 8 November I had this to say:

> *"Some days I just want to cry – not for myself – though life is hard and full on for a carer – but for Marg. I caught her crying quietly to herself, trying for it not to be noticed, when we were having lunch at a café at Carindale. I had been trying, without success, to have her suck through a straw. She had little Emer across the table doing it easily. It gave me an insight into what perhaps she goes through in her own mind. I tend, as I am sure others do, to forget about her feelings and concentrate on my own embarrassment. How un-Jesus like is that!"*

I noticed that if Margaret believed people were looking at her she would not eat. The selection of a table to sit at in public was thus important. She would do best if she was facing me and not the passing parade. At times mirrors were a distraction because there would be her 'friend' and naturally she wanted to converse with her.

Success in eating out was also largely dependent upon my selecting an appropriate food for Margaret. If it was difficult to pick up, she would play with it but not eat. I would often buy food that I could easily cut up into bite sized pieces for her and if necessary feed them to her on a fork. Cups needed to have handles and ones large enough for her to easily hold. I would always ask that her cup be no more than three quarters filled.

So far I had not had much reason to enact the power of attorney we had drawn up. Margaret's name remained on most documents as we usually had all our assets in joint names. This created its own set of problems when people could not or did not choose to understand what it meant to suffer from Alzheimer's disease. I describe one example in my diary of 1 October:

> *"I contacted Energex after doing the floors and some washing. The girl needed to get the OK from Margaret. I should have said*

that I was her attorney but instead said she had Alzheimer's. Still she talked to Marg who was unable to give her name or birth date, etc. I eventually gave all the info. It shook up Margaret for most of the day. She did not know why people asked her these things."

Margaret developed a growing fear that I would put her somewhere. In retrospect I am sure that came from the neurologist's advice to start such a process. In the months of October, November and December I make reference to this fear, one that she based on her sense of being of no use to anyone. So in November she tried to tell me she is okay as long as I am with her. I write on 2 December:

"Marg seemed to be convinced I was going to do something with the house. I sense at times she knows she may have to have care. I tell her she is safe here with me. I will tend to her for as long as God allows me to."

For myself and for the immediate family there were times and events that were hard to accept. In fact to reread some of these affects me deeply again. On 14 January:

"Margaret woke in a better frame of mind I thought. She was more alive, talked and even laughed on occasion. Have to enjoy the good times. By close of day, however, she was a little confused. I don't get so hurt now when she does not know who Vince O'Rourke is. Told me he must be one of my brothers."

How wrong I was to suggest that such things did not hurt. Just two weeks later on 27 January:

"What a sad day — for me that is. I have had a really bad emotional day with Marg. No matter how much my head tells me that Marg is no longer in control of what is going on within her, still I can't control the personal emotional hurt. She does not recognise me as her husband nor does she seem to understand me as father of our children. Thinks I am a nice man whom she likes/loves, but not as her husband. In fact she

> *sees me as different people during the course of the day. Megan rang tonight. I broke down, which I regret. She and the others have enough to cope with."*

As was now common procedure, this confused state went on for quite a few weeks and then it seemed to drop out of her consciousness. I think I dealt with it over the years by choosing to forget about it. Margaret would often talk to me throughout the day about this 'other man' she kept running into in the house. While she would look embarrassed when I told her it was me, she would repeat the story later on in the day. To cap it off, my Margaret always wanted to go home. When I would tell her of this request she would tell me that was news to her. She would look upset that she would ever have wanted to go home.

It was interesting to watch how her mind was working. On 8 April after breakfast she suddenly realised I was Vince. A week or so later just before we rose for the day she told me what she thought Vince was doing and was "surprised that I was Vince." Putting the name to the face was not limited to me. On 20 April Margaret came upstairs to tell me about a person who was downstairs watching the TV. It was our daughter Anne who had called in to visit. Margaret was convinced it could not be Anne. I guess I can now laugh at these incidents, like the time in late August when we had called in to see Megan. While there:

> *"Marg told them about this nasty fellow. She had no idea she was talking about me."*

At least I hoped Margaret did not believe it was me. It did show how sensitive she was to my moodiness. I note on 20 September:

> *"She was in tears when she came out to breakfast. She told me no one loved her. She could not do things. I must admit it made me cry too. I told her how much she is loved by all her family and no more so than by me. She is the centre of my life, now as in the past."*

As the year's end fast approached, I reflected on 27 December, the day after my birthday:

> "Some days I feel that I am in the middle of a distance race and the second wind has not yet kicked in. You feel like you want to stop and sit and relax. Then I ask myself what would Jesus say to me. I think I believe it would be that greater love no one has than they give their life for the other. I am no martyr, I really hate pain, I also am more selfish than selfless, but I know my call at this time is to give my life for Marg even though she does not fully appreciate it."

Nevertheless there were good times. There was also:

> "That beautiful side of her nature whereby she says thanks every time I do something for her."

The carer cannot but be weighed down by the stresses of the job. It may bring some balance to our journey if I sometimes highlight the nicer events that we experienced along the way. It is these events which I found gave me hope and strength. On 6 February:

> "All the family had gathered and I cooked an OK meal thank God. Marg told them all how great it was to have all her loved ones around her. My heart leapt up at how she spoke and her face meant it. I really treasure such moments."

It was her birthday party and, I suggest, the last that she would reasonably participate in. When Margaret was in tune with what was going on around her she would smile a lot and her eyes would sparkle. The deeper the disease, the duller the eyes became. After a visit by her first little granddaughter, Emer, on 9 April:

> "I note the joy in Marg's eyes even though she forgets they were here later on in the day."

At evening mass on 11 May our parish priest, Brendan, asked all the mothers present to come forward for a special mother's day blessing.

> *"Talked Marg into going up front. She was hesitant but went. Thought, by the way, that she was the most beautiful woman there."*

Some mornings I could coax Margaret to sleep a little longer by holding her in my arms. It seemed to make her feel safe and secure like a little child. It was rare for Margaret to initiate a hug, but she did so on 24 August:

> *"Marg woke and really wanted to hug me. It was beautiful. For some reason she sensed I may be going to get rid of her. She told me how much she wanted to be with me. I could have cried."*

There is no doubt in my mind how powerful a force in our lives is love. Our journey was one premised on love.

Chapter 6

2003

Securing Regular Assistance

As I glanced through my diary for 2003, I was acutely aware that every page had comments about our now daily confrontation with aspects of Margaret's disease. It is therefore difficult for me to determine how best to provide a sense of the fullness of the calls upon the carer and the growing dysfunction of the sufferer. The approach I have chosen is to write a month by month overview of events and challenges. This may well lead to some repetition, yet that is exactly what life was like - repetition day after day.

During January Margaret and I continued our walks through the local park. Keeping fit was, I believed, important for our quality of life. Margaret seemed to enjoy the walks although she wanted to sit down and rest more often than she did in 2002. In 2003 she would become very anxious if we deviated in any way from our normal route. She would worry that we may be lost. I would try to convince her that we were not lost and that I could get us back to our starting point. To help in this I would try to keep our car in sight. We drove to the park for our walk. For Margaret's peace of mind, I found that it was necessary to follow the same path each time we went walking in the park.

The importance of Margaret's mirror friend grew:

"Second day of the New Year and already I am wondering how we will get through it all. Marg spends over 50% of her waking hours in this house in front of a large mirror talking to her own image. I almost feel as though I have to excuse myself every time I speak to her because it takes her away from the image. At times when she sees my image in there she will try to walk through the mirror."

I suppose I should have been relieved that Margaret had a 'friend' to talk to, to be with. Yet to accept this type of aberrant behaviour as normal for her in her condition was hard on me, her carer, real friend, and husband.

"I seem to have been through a cycle of emotional traumas today. Began when Marg told me to 'get out' when she was with her image before breakfast. Had to control my reactions. She seemed to be set against me and pals only with her image. Found myself at one stage bent over the sink washing her shirts with tears rolling down my face and my chest heaving in sobs. Throughout the day I could feel the tears well up as I would think of her. I think I want her as she was, keep hoping for that, yet the reality seems so far from that."

I became so upset about the mirror events that I rang the Alzheimer's Association and spoke to a lady about it. Naturally the advice was to leave her be as it was doing her no harm. I initially thought that Margaret related only to the image in the full length mirror. In a while I would notice her speaking to images in every mirror in the house. The most significant outcome from my contact with the Alzheimer's Association was being advised to begin the process of having Margaret assessed, because access to services flowed through such an assessment. Two days later I had need to take Margaret to our family doctor.

"He thinks I must have an assessment done. He noted how much Marg had deteriorated. Reminded me that Aricept plateaus then the drop off is marked."

I finally reached a decision that even if I was to continue as Margaret's carer, I should get whatever help was available to me. On 7 January I rang the Coorparoo Community Services Centre. I was informed that I may well be able to access a Federal Government funded carer's allowance and also gain assistance with providing incontinence aids. The ACAT assessment process was separate. I tried to explain to Margaret what I was doing, but it simply upset her. I told her it was necessary for us to cover all bases just in case I fell ill.

Two social workers came to see us on 13 January. Prior to their coming Margaret was very suspicious about why any of this was necessary. The visit took a good two hours.

> "I was pleased to have both Anne and Megan present. Got emotional once. They were very professional and left me with hope of help in the future. They have followed up seeking help with OT (occupational therapist) issues and the ACAT process. Latter could take 6 months. Megan told me that Marg yesterday cried and told her she wished she were perfect again. Been a long and emotionally draining day."

I did apply for the carer's allowance on 16 January and received a letter from Centrelink saying my application was successful. That letter arrived on 28 January. The next day I received from the State Government a disability parking permit that our family doctor had suggested we apply for. On its receipt:

> "I was pleased and yet it weighs heavily on me to think of her as one who is disabled."

I cannot speak highly enough of the support I received from the Coorparoo Community Services Centre. They rang me on 24 January to check on how I was going. They had left me a couple of incontinence pads to try out and now would send me another sample. To find one that was better for control and still comfortable for Margaret was a process of trial and error.

The Centre staff did also advise me to make contact with a support group. I admit I never did. It may have been my nature to say I don't need that level of support or it may be part of being the typical Aussie male. I believe though that I would have benefited from hearing first hand how others were dealing with similar situations, particularly when the carer was a male caring for a woman. I was chuffed that the Centre's representative:

> "Told me that I should be proud of what I am doing for Margaret."

I would hear that said on a number of occasions. I could not begin to imagine not so caring for the love of my life. Megan, our second daughter, began to spend time with her mother to give me a little break. She would try to involve Margaret in art type activities. For example, they would paint wooden tissue boxes and then decorate them with various transfers. Margaret loved this diversion. We gave some of the decorated boxes to family members on their birthdays. I could never seem to find the time for such activities. I am sure Margaret would have loved more diversionary activities than the few I was able to provide.

On 9 January it was obvious that my Margaret was no longer behaving in a manner normally associated with her chronological age. It was incumbent upon me to try to understand where she was in her new time frame.

> "A change today was to watch Marg talk to Raggie Anne Doll, the little pup and the teddy as real things. I was bemused but did not let it get to me. Later she and Megan named the dog 'Sam'. I only hope she will let the kids play with them."

Margaret was very possessive of these few items. She would become very upset when any of the grandchildren took them to play with whenever they were visiting our home.

Toileting was becoming more and more difficult now that Margaret could not take herself when nature called. As I mentioned before, it was the case that if I remained calm, not an easy thing for me, Margaret also remained calm no matter the problem. If I reacted aggressively, she would react as violently as my gentle wife was capable. Night was a problem period due to the number of times we were both up. As a consequence, lack of sleep would affect our behaviours during the day.

In terms of general care Margaret was hardest to manage in the mornings and again by mid afternoon. At breakfast she would often forget what she was about, walk away to do other things and I would have to convince her to come back to finish her meal. At other times she ate reasonably well, although she would often have trouble eating her sandwiches at lunch. With encouragement she could cope. She was now an expert at hiding her tablets in her mouth while drinking water to wash them down. She had started this practice in 2002.

> *"I have just given up on trying to encourage Marg to swallow her vitamin E capsule. She puts it between her teeth and the side of her mouth, drinks any amount of water and cannot understand it needs to be swallowed. I get so aggro but I may as well be talking to the wall. She on her part begins to dislike taking tablets. Perhaps it is time to drop it out of her tablet regime. The frustration just is not worth it."*

Margaret was now totally reliant on my assistance with almost every aspect of her personal life. I was growing in stature as a hair stylist and manicurist. At least I thought so. I seldom gave much thought as to what all this meant to Margaret and then on 17 January I gained some insight into her inner thoughts.

> *"When we were at breakfast Marg began to cry. She sometimes seemed scared when routine is broken. Anne had arrived for me to take the car in for its service. Funny how different is the morning. Before she went to sleep last night she talked to me – almost coherently – about her terrible illness, her fears, her wish to be well and that she loved me and thanked me for being so good to her. I could have cried. Then today when we walked down to pick up the car she said to me in the car, 'Who are you? One of the boys?' She told me she knew I was Vince her husband only after I told her."*

Margaret would often keep looking at me as if I were a complete stranger. I found this one of the most difficult aspects of the disease to deal with emotionally. Nevertheless, there were times which were quite a contrast as on her birthday, 7 February:

> "Had a great birthday for Marg today. She is 64. Her eyes were alive and sparkling tonight. I can't remember seeing her so alive, within reason of course. She really loved having the family around, being the centre of attention. She did not try to extract herself. She did, at one stage, ask me how she was to get home. Marg got some lovely gifts. When I read her cards to her she cried. Sometimes I wonder just how much gets through to her. She is the love of my life always."

Life was always full of little dramas. Later in the month when we were preparing to go to mass she hid my church money. I could not find it anywhere. When we were at mass, Margaret again received communion and carried it back to her seat where I had to convince her to eat it. That evening she refused to eat her meal. All of this was par for the course on any one day. I often thought that some of Margaret's ways had to be seen for their humour to add balance to life.

> "When we are eating she can't wait to get up and move off. Says she will come back but never does. She keeps talking to tea towels too and hiding them. Seem to spend a lot of my day seeking items. She has no idea where they now are."

After a time I would grow to know where they were most likely to be hidden. Our old Queenslander home had many nooks and crannies for hiding. Her favourite places included under pillows and cushions. Items that could be folded were always neatly folded before they were hidden away.

During the month of February I continued to seek outside assistance. On 4 February two representatives from the Coorparoo Community Services Centre visited:

> "They wanted information so we can get a free supply of incontinence pads for Marg. Told it would take up to 6 months to start the process."

The process required that I obtain a letter from our family doctor. The doctor felt that not everything that could be done had been done in Margaret's case and suggested she try another tablet that may alleviate the problem. He was totally correct in his call that not everything available had been tried. However, rightly or wrongly, I felt let down:

> "Angry I guess that there is no real understanding from our side. What pill can help Margaret find the toilet in time, or help her to recall how to undress to sit on the toilet and so on? I said buggar them, we will buy our own pads."

My frustration grew when I had noted in my diary that an Occupational Therapist was to visit from DAART, a domiciliary acute care and rehabilitation service, on 12 February at 9.30am. When no one turned up, I rang only to find that they had no record of the proposed visit. They promised to ring me back. I did not receive a return call. I bit my tongue and rang DAART again on 13 February. Once again I was told that I could expect a return call that day. Again no return call was made. I wondered at times whether the lack of urgency was related to my being a male trying to work through what I saw as a 'woman's problem' – incontinence pads for women.

Help came for me when my contact from the Coorparoo Community Services Centre rang me about the letter I was supposed to obtain from our family doctor. I could always count on their support.

> "Told her of my run in about that. She would try to get us on the list without it. No promises though. Also explained about DAART. She was to ring for me. Got a call back to say a representative would be here on Monday."

Indeed the OT did come on 17 February and her assistance was much appreciated. She suggested a number of changes including grab rails for the shower, taking off the sliding shower door, a rail in the toilet and a temperature control for the hot water system. She would arrange for a body called Home Assist Secure to assist with all the changes. A bloke from Home Assist came on the 25 February:

> "He will arrange for a tradesman to put the rails etc in

> *the bathroom. Because we get a carer's allowance from the Commonwealth he is able to have the government fund the labour. We need to meet the cost of the rails etc. It looks like a good service we can call upon over time."*

The work was completed the next day. Margaret initially had difficulty using the grab rails. It was the same with anything new. She never did get used to the hand rail in the toilet. I found that having only a curtain on the shower instead of a sliding glass door made helping Margaret, while she was showering, much easier.

I had read about sleep deprivation being used as a form of torture. I wondered how that would work. More so than before, I was now experiencing its effects and would do so for a number of years ahead. My diaries are filled with references to lack of sleep and the mood swings both of us experienced as a result.

As I reflect on our journey I realise that I had kept us in the one bed for too long. I may well have had more sleep if we had moved to single beds sooner. I also realise that I was slow, too slow and too proud, to take the offers made by my daughters to give me a night off once in a while. Every carer needs to have adequate sleep if at all possible - just ask mothers of young children.

In the past we would have been up at least once every night. During 2003 every night was punctuated with a number of wakeful periods. Margaret would grow agitated and wake. Once awake she would either sit up or try to exit the bed. I would have to assume that she had a need to visit the toilet. I was thankful if we woke only twice a night. Three times was the average, though some nights were like that of the 16 February:

> *"Had a broken night. Went to bed at 10.15 or so. Could not go to sleep. Up at 11.30, 12.30, 2.15, 3.30 and 4.25 or so, then again at 6.30. Makes a difference to how you feel."*

I read somewhere that Valerian may help with regulating sleep. We tried it, but it really had little effect for Margaret. Later I would try Melatonin which, I believe, was a little better, though it was so diluted in its tablet form that one would need to take the whole bottle of tablets for it to make a real difference. Most books published in the USA that I read suggested its use for the

Alzheimer sufferer. In the United States it was not diluted to the extent that it was in Australia. Finally, I found that tenderness and care were the most effective tools. After being awake beyond midnight on 21 February:

> *"Put her to bed, left the light on out on the verandah, said our prayers together then I cradled her in my arms, stroked her forehead and hair. She asked me to look after her and said, 'I love you'. It took 10 minutes before her eyes closed then 45 minutes to go to sleep. She twitched violently throughout. I can cry even now as I recall it. What she suffers is not to be belittled."*

We would try this method often and, though it worked, I eventually sought and bought some mild sleeping tablets for Margaret. I tried to capture how I was seeing our existence on 28 February:

> *"Life at the moment seems to me to be a series of days of pain - some worse than others - with a sprinkle of the absence of pain."*

When I did give Margaret a sleeping tablet on 1 March it knocked her right out. She almost fell off the toilet at 1.30am. I decided to use them only as a last resort. I discussed the use of the tablets with one of the Coorparoo Community Services Centre staff when she rang to speak to me on 4 March. I was pleased to learn that the tablets took effect usually for between 4 to 6 hours. Margaret could have a whole or half a tablet even as late as 1am if necessary. In the end I hardly ever used the tablets, which may well have been too conservative an approach.

As mentioned earlier lack of sleep, broken sleep, was simply now an aspect of daily life. Tongue in cheek I suggested in one of my diaries that I keep mentioning lack of sleep:

> *"Because it probably helps me feel better when I get cranky with her during the day."*

Of course there were variations to consider. For a few months Margaret would get out of bed and wander around the house.

> "Put Marg to bed about 10. She looked tired. She was up walking around soon after and I had a devil of a job getting her back to bed at 11.15. Almost got to the point of turning out the lights and leaving her wander. She was still restless and awake at 12.30. I decided to give her a sleeping tablet. It worked well until 6.30."

Part of the explanation for Margaret's inability to get to sleep was that she would often have a little nap in the lounge chair during the day. Once in bed she seemed to prefer to lie on her back and hence would snore. Her snoring would then force me to move to one of the other rooms and I never found it easy to sleep well in a foreign bed. In my thoughts expressed in my diary of 13 March I try to indicate how deeply tiredness and frustration can affect the carer:

> "I suppose I don't want to fully express it, but there are times, today is one, when I wish either Marg would come back to me as I remember her, or she would be taken from me quickly. The emotional drain is probably harder to bear than the physical. I still love and respect her so deeply, yet there is little even recognition in return. She really is a little child (baby) in adult form with no prospect of growing out of that childhood, rather will she further regress. God, forgive such thoughts."

On this day my daughter Megan spent a fair amount of the day with Margaret taking her to the doctor and visiting Margaret's mother. She rang me the next day:

> "Seems she had been reflecting on her day with Marg yesterday. It gave her a rare insight into what my own days must really be like, let alone how Marg feels. I was uplifted by the fact that someone now has that insight."

I would still try to get Margaret to go for a walk with me during the day. We would also go out somewhere each morning. Her reaction remained constant i.e. wanted to go out, enjoyed the outing for 45 minutes or so then wanted to go home, and then once home:

> "She often treats me with reserve and seems to not want to be there."

Margaret could be moody depending upon how disturbed her sleep had been that night. She also had an ability to hide all manner of things. You had to laugh at times. We had bought some fresh fish for tea. When we reached home I asked Marg to take the fish upstairs for me while I locked the garage and took out the rubbish bins:

> "The fish disappeared. Looked everywhere for 15 minutes. Marg had no idea where it was. Eventually with the help of St Anthony I found it in the upstairs pedal rubbish bin."

These occasions call for a sense of humour from the carer. Margaret could show signs of a sense of humour too:

> "Marg gave me a laugh last night. I said to her, 'roll over baby boo please'. Half asleep she replied, 'Okay daddy.' Then she giggled."

The day before this she had showed her caring side. We had been shopping:

> "I left Marg at the car to put the trolley in its bay and she, beautiful dear, came after me offering her hand to show me to the car. Even now her nature is to look after others."

I believe that Margaret's 'turns' returned during this month. They did seem to be less frequent.

> "After dressing, before breakfast, she got very pale. I thought she would faint. Gave her a drink and she lay down until breakfast. She has been rather 'remote' all day. Her conversation is even less rational and still looks pale. My heart races at these times wondering what will happen next."

With the benefit of hindsight this particular incident could have been the result of Margaret not taking her blood pressure tablets. The tablet was large. It was one of those she would hide in her mouth only to take out and hide after I had left her. I found 6 or 7 of them one day hidden in a dark recess between two cabinets. Towards the end of the month Megan bought me a good mortar and pestle to grind up such tablets. I could now ground those tablets that were suitable, mix them in honey or jam and then give them to Margaret. There was a need to approach both our doctor and our pharmacist to ensure the tablets could be ground before taking them. In one case we had to change to a different tablet, as the one she was taking was of the slow release type.

Of great interest to me in rereading my diary for March is the discovery of an event I had completely forgotten. It happened on 15 March:

> *"At breakfast Marg suddenly complained of pain in her left shoulder. Her eyes were wide. I though of heart but checked the shoulder as it is often sore each day. There was a swelling the size of half a tennis ball."*

Our family doctor believed it had bled into the muscle. We used cold packs. The swelling was still noticeable a week later so we arranged an X-ray on 25 March. There was no bone damage and it was thought that it could have been a flare up of Margaret's rheumatoid arthritis. Just to add to this month's events we both came down with severe head colds.

As a carer you are often learning as you go. Experience is truly a great teacher and in my case much of the learning came out of bad experiences. So when I found it too difficult to have Margaret move off her back at night, I would go to the nearby bedroom. Ultimately I would fall asleep and sleep very deeply. On returning to our bedroom I came to realise how important it was to regularly check on Margaret's condition. She would often be bladder incontinent throughout the night. I also learned a lot about the absorbency of various types of incontinence pads. No amount of reading of labels was as useful as experience.

I have found that the carer has to become adept at reading body language. Agitation after or during meals usually indicated a need for toileting. I am sure mothers can relate well to this requirement in raising small children. Just as the child may wander away to some private place so too would my Alzheimer's sufferer. To force the issue of using the toilet when I thought it was required failed. Even standing beside my Margaret to encourage her did not work. How I ever expected it to work I just don't know now, but desperation drives you to do strange things. What I failed to comprehend, as I struggled with incontinence, was the need for a regular routine, a need I did not address for some time.

Dealing with faecal incontinence was definitely the most difficult aspect of my role as carer. I am ashamed as I look back at the number of times I treated my beautiful wife so poorly in dealing with such incontinence.

> *"While at times I wonder if a God of love really exists, at other times I wonder how that God, if existing, will deal with me. I treat Marg quite badly at times. Today for the fifth day she soiled herself after lunch sometime. This no matter how often I have asked her to use the toilet. I can even sit her on it and she will point blankly refuse to use it. Then later she will go but only after partly soiling herself. She always denies the evidence. I get annoyed, yell at times, call her names, almost I am in tears. Yet she has to just remain patient though afraid of my tantrum while I bath her and refresh her, wash her clothes, the shower, etc. Later she will fuss over me and wonder what it is I am so annoyed about. I see nothing but goodness in her as I have always done. She is now so simple, so reliant, so open to abuse without recrimination. God please help me in my weakness."*

Bladder incontinence was seldom a problem during the day. I can't say the same thing for faecal incontinence though. I found that if I set myself deliberately at the start of the day to remain calm no matter the number of incidents I had to attend to; I could generally be true to that. The one day at a time approach has great merit. However, I could find a lot of reasons for not adhering to the process which was my undoing.

Help was close at hand, thank God. My daughter, Megan, had followed up my request for an ACAT assessment. The assessment was to be held on 16 April. I was also informed that

I was now on the list for support from MASS with respect to a supply of incontinence pads.

The ACAT assessment took the better part of 2 hours.

> *"She asked Marg a lot of questions and got weird responses, but it showed how far Marg's cognitive ability had declined. She does an assessment then takes it to her Board. Says Marg is in the High Need category. Counselled me that I was not created to kill myself for Marg and leave her alone – the carer must take care also. She will recommend Marg for long term respite, for CAPS, for day care, etc. Some I can take my time about. One thing is for sure that I will not be able to do everything forever. Gave a lot of practical advice and insights into memory loss, eating habits, safety and security. Praised us for the level of care we have already given. Megan was present. Anne came later. What a family I am blest with."*

By the next day Glenda, who carried out the ACAT assessment the day before, advised me she had referred Margaret to St Luke's for in-home care. Their representative would visit us in the following week. On 24 April:

> *"Today a lovely young lady from St Luke's arrived about 10.30. She took a lot of notes as usual. They offer a wide range of services and will start with 2 by 2 hours a week in-house respite for me. When we see how Marg and I handle that we can look to other things. She also told us how good a job I am doing and how great to have a family helping. She said I must look after myself if I am going to be able to look after Marg."*

I was in desperate need of help yet I was slow to take up an offer for other than the minimum available. I regret that. If I could offer one piece of strong advice to all carers it would be to be sure to care for yourself. Each carer's aim is to look after the one needing the care, but the carer can only offer the best service if they are relaxed, well rested, healthy, and strong physically, emotionally and socially. The carer is the greatest asset in the life of the one suffering. Please, look after the asset.

Towards the end of the month I took ill. I was very ill for about three days. My family was my safety net otherwise I hate to think of poor Margaret's lot at this time. Margaret worried about me:

> "Poor dear, Marg would caress my hair; tell me how she did not want to lose me. Her mothering is alive and well."

The family were my strength:

> "At times like this one is reminded of the great gift of family where family is loving and caring. I can almost reach out and touch the love and concern. It is a beautiful feeling, so safe and secure in its own way."

Notwithstanding our daily struggles we continued to go for walks and I took Margaret into the city by bus. She thoroughly enjoyed the experience especially when we caught up with Maree and Emer for a cuppa. She always enjoyed her time with the kids. A few weeks later she would likewise enjoy a day out with the grandchildren eating fish and chips on the foreshore at Wynnum.

Easter was always a special time for us as a family. We would gather to celebrate Passover together at the home of Maree and Michael. This year was no exception. Margaret enjoyed the evening and on the way home she talked her head off about someone that even she could willingly kill. I have no idea how that came out of a Passover celebration other than on the news there had been a lot about Saddam Hussein. I think he was the one she had in mind.

One of my lasting images comes on 26 April.

> "After tea Marg disappeared. I later found her in our bedroom. She had pulled all the buttons off her red cardigan. Where there were buttons there were large holes in the wool. She had begun to pull them off her shirt too. I lost it. Told her I would put her in a home, etc. She denied she had done it. I think her 'image' did it. Rang Maree to offload. She was great. Told me mum was worth more than $40 for a cardigan. Calmed me down I

> *guess until the next time. Trying to find reasons for the non-reasoning is futile. God love her."*

This would not be the last such episode. I have often tried to pull buttons off shirts and have failed. I can now only guess at the mental anguish and frustration that would cause one to tug and tug until the buttons came off. It certainly forced me to hone my skills in darning and re-buttoning. I am ever thankful for the 6 months at boarding school and being taught to knit and sew by the nuns at Koongal in Rockhampton.

Every six weeks I took Margaret to the hairdresser. I noticed Mary watching Margaret having an animated conversation with her image in one of the many mirrors. What I loved about Mary was that she just continued on and spoke with Margaret as she always had done. By the end of May though, we discussed whether or not to continue to dye Margaret's hair. The length of time taken was a problem. Mary very generously offered to come to our home if and when that became necessary.

May brought cooler weather and so Margaret slept a little better, though lack of sleep combined with incontinence were still our major concern. It would be that way until Margaret entered a nursing home. Margaret would very often wake and indicate a need to go to the toilet between 3 and 4am. Getting Margaret back to sleep after that was far from easy. It was obvious that I needed to change her routine. I can say that to change her routine was, for me, almost impossible.

The aid I was now receiving from St Luke's was most welcome. If I had a concern initially, it was that I simply did not know exactly when the aide would arrive. Eventually we reached an agreement that we would try a four hour stint on one morning each fortnight. I think the organisers at St Luke's were afraid that, if we did not have an agreement, I would grow frustrated and eventually refuse their help. My impatience I put down to my Irish grandparents.

I have said before, but it bears repeating, our time together after tea was the best time of the day. When a carer finds a time like that, be sure to use it well. On 23 May:

> *"Marg told me she likes sitting with me watching TV. It must*

be quite a change from all the time she spends talking to herself in the mirrors."

Talking to her mirror image became a more public issue. On 20 June while we were shopping at Carindale:

"She waved, smiled, said hello to herself in a mirror. I try not to look too embarrassed."

At the beginning of June I began to seek more help for dealing with Margaret's incontinence. I had previously found talking to nurses via the National Incontinence Hotline was invaluable. I now sought to discuss it with one of the staff from St Luke's. They arranged for a nurse to visit me within a week. Meantime, I had received a letter suggesting it was again time for Margaret to have her regular mammogram. I rang and explained Margaret's condition and it was agreed that the process would be too difficult for her. The way forward should any problems arise may be the use of an ultrasound examination.

The nurse from St Luke's arrived on 5 June:

"She was a delightful lady. Said I was open for 4 hours support each week. No need to go to Grey Power as St Luke's can give me the housework support I need. She will suggest, on my request, one hour a fortnight as a starting point. We talked about incontinence. Said it was normal to find cleaning up distasteful. Only real suggestion was to be firm about trying to set a toilet regime after breakfast. Need for patience."

I certainly was slow to take up the offer of help. I believed that help with housework would be the most beneficial help for me. We were self funded retirees. Such beings are not all the same. There are those that just fall over the line into that category and those that far exceed the line. We just fell over the line. I mention this as there was a greater array of assistance if you were a pensioner. We would have to pay a nominal amount for many of the services provided. It would be money well spent. In my case Centrelink's carers allowance just about covered our cost for assistance. I often wondered how many thousands of dollars we saved the government.

I tried to be rather stern with Margaret about remaining in the toilet after breakfast. In this way I began to see a slight improvement. In fact within weeks I would have to let her know that it was okay to leave, just as you might to a young child. Furthermore, I started to realise how important it was to come to understand Margaret's patterns. After meals was an obvious time to try, but that did not work regularly. It was the exception for Margaret to toilet herself. Even when she did so, like the little child, she needed help with cleaning. Constipation had the effect of making me even more watchful and concerned. At such times I would try exercise and more fruit in our diet. The other end of the spectrum can be left to the imagination.

I firmly believe that there is no substitute for having a regular regime even though there will still be mishaps. It made such a vast difference to the quality of both our lives when we had days without incontinence. Persistence together with patience would appear to be the keys.

On 10 June the first carer from St Luke's came to the house. She was younger than I expected and I was amazed that:

"Margaret introduced herself by name."

I was not sure that the younger woman and Margaret would be a successful mix.

"This was a get to know you visit. They did some painting. Don't think Marg likes having to do things all the time. Seems we are set down for 3 hours on Tuesdays."

I formed the opinion that three hours may be excessive to begin with. I was the insecure one and the one who had a routine in place as I look back. St Luke's and I discussed the level of support on 16 June and we agreed to change to four hours each fortnight. They did not have personnel to help with house work at that time.

The carer from St Luke's came at 8am on 24 June. I later had that time changed as I could not get Margaret up, clothed and toileted after breakfast by 8am. Before the carer arrived Margaret had one of her 'turns'.

> "At breakfast Marg looked pale. She talked about babies and a woman who did not want her there."

Actually I wondered whether she and the mirror image had had a falling out. The four hours did allow me to have a haircut, go to a café, visit my daughter, etc. I was still concerned as to how Margaret would relate to the particular carer. I would find out at the next visit on 8 July. I used the time to squeeze in a game of golf but:

> "Rushed home when Anne indicated all had not gone well. Anne tells me Marg gave her carer a hard time. She told her she should not be here at all. Wanted her to leave the house. I can't get over her being that way. Perhaps it is because the carer looks so young. Gave Marg a good tea and she seemed settled. Has no knowledge of the events or so she says."

I followed this up with St Luke's. Seems they rang the carer on our home phone while she was with Margaret. Margaret reacted violently to this young person using her phone. She actually struck the carer. This was so out of character though the books about Alzheimer's will warn about the potential for this disease to change people's behaviours. In the wash up a more senior carer was assigned to Margaret. Problems would still arise, but by and large Margaret reacted more calmly to someone more mature. It must be difficult to match the carer to the client.

As in every month, indeed every week, there were some good times not to be forgotten. I would on occasion take Margaret out with me to the golf range. She would sit and pretend to read while I vainly tried to hit the balls. Going out regularly for a morning coffee or visiting her mother and/or our children and grandchildren were always good times.

We took a three day holiday to the coast. Our daughter Anne came with us once again thank God. We had booked an apartment sight unseen and stayed there just for one night. It simply did not suit our needs. The toilet door opened inward which made it very difficult for me to help Margaret. We inspected a couple of alternative places and made a move.

Prior inspection is, I think, a necessity. There could be any number of things for different persons to consider. We had a specific requirement. As I have mentioned, Margaret's 'friend' was her mirror image. Many holiday units have many mirrors in the toilet / bathroom area. Margaret would not sit on a toilet if her 'friend' was there with her. At one time I had to hang a sheet over the mirrors as the only way to have her use the facility.

Margaret grew to have some new 'people' in her life. I think I have mentioned the few dolls she befriended. Now I found that she had one of a group of pillows on the lounge chairs she would play with throughout the day. She would speak to it as if speaking to a child. She would cover it to make it comfortable and sit beside it. In fact, I would coax her to sit at times just to relieve the strain on her back from leaning over the chair for so long. At times Margaret would upset her granddaughter by not allowing her to play with or jump on her 'baby'.

Though I do not want to pillory myself, I am embarrassed to admit that I could never totally control my emotional outbursts in the face of Margaret's incontinence. It was always the one issue that would set me off no matter how much I tried to remain calm. I confessed after cleaning up my beautiful wife on 17 June:

> *"The anger rose - angry at what? - the clean up, my embarrassment for her, my hatred for the fact she cannot, will not, use the toilet even though I know her reasoning is all but non existent. I ranted and raved and even struck her on the backside like I would a child. What fear did that cause her, what insecurity, yet trapped in this house with me whom she does not recognise as her husband of 37 or more years. I cleaned her. Later apologised and, like the saint she has always been, forgave me and told me I was a lovely man. God forgive me, Vince forgive yourself."*

I can admit now that I am not sure to this day if I have really forgiven myself for raising my hand to one so loved, loving and vulnerable. My diary notes indicate very clearly that whenever I asked my Margaret for forgiveness she always forgave, and then showed concern for me and my wellbeing. What makes me feel worse about my intolerance was that our family doctor had said to me on 4 July that:

> "I need to understand that the connection between the head and bowel is not working, hence the incontinence."

And further:

> "In the end it will be too much for me to care for her myself"

I hated hearing that, but deep down I knew it to be realistic. I dreaded the day that I might have to give my love into the care of others.

It seemed that Margaret suffered yet another 'turn' on 23 July:

> "Found her looking into the distance at one stage. She told me there was something wrong in her head and she did not know what she should do. God I hate this disease."

I reflected on our needs the next night:

> "If God is testing me, He is doing a great job and I am failing more often than not. I had a feeling at one stage today that Marg felt so alone. I wondered what it must be like for her, so I hugged her and kissed her hair. She said, "Thank you" three times. I just wish I could keep in focus her needs not my inconvenience etc. I think to be able to put the other first, almost without thinking, must be what sainthood is about."

Some days later we had dinner with Maree, Michael and family. Margaret always had a special love for Maree's husband, Michael. He was so kind and gentle with her she reacted positively. It was little Emer's three and one third birthday. Any excuse for a party would do. Margaret enjoyed herself immensely, so much so that I write on the next day:

> "I am still up about how well Marg seemed to enjoy the night out last night. She sang, she danced, she smiled and really enjoyed herself."

Such moments are the priceless pearl days and should be treasured as such. They occurred very infrequently. When they did, it was as if a veil was lifted from Margaret's diseased brain for a short time. The pity of it was that she could not recall it in a short space of time. She loved her grandchildren so deeply, and yet the pleasure that comes from being fully a grandmother to them was denied her. We do, thank God, have a pictorial record of Margaret showing her holding each of her five grandchildren at some stage.

No matter how intellectually I realised there would be no cure for this disease, I would leap at anything that proposed a betterment of Margaret's quality of life. Thus during August and September I put my trust in a new drug called Ebixa. My sister Helen had heard a report about it on the radio. I could recall our local pharmacist telling me of it too. It was not on the Government's support list but it sounded rather promising.

If I am correct in my memory it was a drug that may help in elongating the process, but did not suggest a cure. Interestingly for me, it could be taken in conjunction with the other medication Margaret was already taking. I would not again take Margaret off her Aricept. It was new enough that our family doctor needed to make enquiries about it. We thought there was little to lose in trying it. A month's supply cost me $158 and that was not the dearest price in the country at that time.

What we would again come to experience is just how differently each person reacts to drugs. I have no doubt this drug will be of great use to others, but let me outline our experience for what that is worth for others.

Margaret began taking the drug on 15 August and two days later:

> *"It may not be the new tablets but Marg has been very vague today. Even stands and stares wondering what to do. I hope it gets better rather than worse."*

By 20 August Margaret was complaining of problems in her head. She began to wander off by herself at times as if trying to go somewhere.

Securing Regular Assistance

> *"Seems not to know what she is / should be doing. I can only put it down to the effects of Ebixa. That is her only new medication."*

But then I began to see signs of hope by 27 August.

> *"I hope the signs I am seeing are that the drug Ebixa is working. She has no trouble combing her hair, some sentences almost make sense, she found her own way back to bed in the dark last night, etc. She was really good looking after Thomas today. She even did one of her crazy dances for him to make him laugh. Calls Michael 'love'."*

The roller coaster ride we were on is indicated in my diary for 2 September:

> *"I am not sure what is going on in Marg at the moment. I get the impression that maybe the Ebixa, the only change in medicines, has awakened parts that were asleep. She seems more conscious that she does not know what she is doing or why she is. She tends to cry more, even crying today - albeit silently - while we were in the butcher shop. Rather embarrassing I must admit. Both yesterday and today she has gotten very annoyed with me when I am trying to give her a shower. Got really angry today. Of course I react badly as if she is doing this rationally. She is talking to herself more too - at least to her image whenever she sees it. The pillow downstairs get a good talking to also - seems it will not do as it is told."*

There was now a new found aggression and severe agitation in Margaret. It reared its head while we were at the hairdresser's salon. She did not want to stay and objected to anyone touching her other than Mary. I was glad to be there to control her. Margaret would now get very cross with me when I took her to the toilet. It was as if the Ebixa had put her back to how she was several months before. We had to go through a rerun as it were and it was very distressing for us both. So by 7 October:

> *"Marg has really been confused - tells me something strange is going on in her mind. She told Megan she wanted to go home*

and the people here for father's day wanted to kill her. When I take her to the toilet she cries while there."

When I left Margaret with Megan the next day it was a disaster. Margaret grew angry and tried to walk out. She would pace about the house like a caged tiger. Luckily Megan had locked all the external doors. In her desperation, Megan decided to take Margaret for a short drive. Somehow she got her mother into the car which was made all the more difficult as she had a small baby to look after. The drive did seem to settle her. I too found that to take her for a short walk outside the house would settle her. On my return she did calm down a little, but not entirely. I did not look forward to the afternoon showering exercise anymore.

Margaret's personality had changed dramatically and quickly. Every adult member of our family recognised and commented on the change. I found the mental and emotional strain of caring for her in this state was wearing me out. It was as if she were taking 'angry pills'. She would turn on her daughters; she would storm away from me and told me very clearly that:

"She no longer wanted to be with me"

She tried to exit via the locked front door. A little later she would calm down. Finally I rang our neurologist to discuss this with him.

"Told me changes could be the disease itself or drug related. Objective fact could be established if gave up Ebixa for 3 weeks to see if any change. Again suggested I look to the long term."

We were no longer visiting the neurologist since, in all our views, it put too much of a strain on Margaret and he was quite definite in his diagnosis.

I decided to call the Alzheimer's Association. The drug was so new that my feedback was the first that they had received. There was no noticeable improvement in Margaret's personality by the end of the month so I dropped the drug out of her medicine regime. Life for us soon returned to what it was prior to our experiment with Ebixa. I do not regret the trial, just the fact that for Margaret this particular drug was not of great benefit either to herself or to me as carer. I wrote on 30 October:

> *"I have noticed a very marked change in her general behaviour since giving up Ebixa. She can still change in moods but seems less stressed in herself."*

During this period we were allocated a different carer for Margaret by St Luke's. She was a delightful person who, no matter what occurred, always seemed calm. I think her age made her more acceptable to Margaret. That did not mean that there were no hiccups.

Whenever there was anyone or anything new to be experienced I would find myself being very anxious and on my guard. I just could not predict how Margaret would react. Rosalie arrived for her first four hour session on 12 August. I stayed around for some time before leaving them and was pleasantly surprised that they hit it off so well together on this first occasion. When Rosa returned in two weeks all went well again. I think it helped that Rosa had a:

> *"Lovely calm way of talking to Marg."*

It may well have been as a result of the Ebixa, but on 16 September I returned home to find my Margaret in a filthy mood with Rosa. Within 30 minutes of my return she had settled again. I did have some concern for the future. A fortnight later:

> *"Marg got very agitated when Rosa arrived. Cried, etc. They could do little. I eventually went out for 30 minutes."*

This was to be my 'sacred' four hours of relief. I would usually organise myself to try to get a number of small jobs done in that time. Any disruption would mean trying to find alternative ways to get to the dentist, doctor, pay bills etc. My own experience was that Margaret was more malleable in the morning. I therefore requested that we change Rosa from coming of an afternoon to the morning. St Luke's obliged by 28 October.

> "They went off in the car. I had tried to tell Marg it was an outing day for her. Rosa reported it went well. They walked for a short time, had a coffee, drove around and visited a shop or two. When they got back home Marg was a bit angry. Did not want to go in upstairs, so I will need to get a set of downstairs' keys. I was very pleased it went well."

The disease certainly does affect moods. It should not have been surprising then that Margaret grew very angry with Rosa when Rosa had to use our toilet. Margaret:

> "Grew red in the face and told Rosa to get out of her house."

Once more this was so far removed from Margaret's normal pattern of behaviour.

I found that I needed to, as it were, 'prime' Margaret prior to her respite carer coming. If I did that and actually walked down to the car with her she would appear more at ease. She did expect often that I would be going with them. To alleviate the anger Margaret would show if Rosa tried to enter the house on their return, Rosa would simply sit outside the door under cover until my return.

As time went on Margaret seemed to grow more definite about not wanting to willingly accept care from anyone other than myself. On 9 December for example I almost had to force her into the car and when she returned with Rosa:

> "She told Rosa she was no longer needed and would not let her come in. Rosa locked Marg in and waited."

Nothing is straight forward in the life of the carer of one suffering from Alzheimer's. Rosa rang me later in the week to discuss how best to deal with Margaret's behaviour on returning home from their outings. I undertook to ensure that I would be at home before them. So on 16 December:

> "Rosa came and took off with a reluctant Margaret. Rosa told me they had a good time together for 2 hours then it was time to head home. I made sure I was home when they arrived and

> *I witnessed the change in Marg towards Rosa once home. She bottled it up though because I was present."*

After some months of trial and error the respite period was working reasonably well. Whenever there was a threat of a change of rosters I would grow very anxious. One thing that was so obvious to me was that the person with Alzheimer's found great difficulty dealing with change. I would always have something to say and I was pleased that St Luke's tried to accommodate our needs.

During the second half of 2003 I was so desperate for assistance I sought and gained help from three other sources. I think that finally the penny was dropping. I was not superman, and 24 hour daily care is not possible for the one person over a long period in which lack of sleep is a norm. St Luke's help was very welcomed as too was the support at various times from my three daughters, my two sisters Helen and Colleen, and also that from Margaret's mother Bernie. Nonetheless I was faltering. There was so much to do each day. As I look back I cannot but be amazed that I was able to cope for so long. The human will is a powerful force as I am sure every carer knows.

On 3 September I was visited by a representative from Ozcare. I had approached them as St Luke's were not able, at that time, to offer me the help I so desperately needed with house work.

> *"The interview process was as we have been through before. I am sure Marg understands parts - enough to storm out towards the end. Thank God Megan was there with us. I may get 3 hours of respite a week from them at $12 per fortnight."*

On 12 September our first Ozcare person arrived. The program was Government subsidised and required that Margaret assist in some way. The carer who came was Janine.

> *"She was really nice to Margaret. She tried to get Marg to help her a little with housework. By and large she did housework ....Marg thought she was OK as long as she could wander."*

Both Margaret and I could not leave the house together if

we wanted our Ozcare person to remain. I can well understand that being the case. I ensured that we did not have appointments requiring our going out together when our Ozcare helper came. We had several Ozcare personnel at home during the next few weeks of the program. Margaret was taking Ebixa and that did not help in her accepting so many different faces. I can imagine that her mood was not helped either by having to accept another woman into her home to do housework. Such was hers to do all our married life. It was one thing for her to accept my doing the work but quite another to accept an outsider, especially another woman.

By November I was really feeling the effects of lack of sleep. On November 11 Rosa from St Luke's talked with me about seeking night-time respite. She gave me several contact numbers. On woman rang me that afternoon and I noted:

> *"I must also look to day respite care. I hate all this but know I must recharge myself if I am to go the journey with Marg. Tears well up every time I think of any of this. Feel I am betraying her trust in me."*

On the same day our family doctor once more warned me to think seriously about institutional care for Margaret. Respite I hoped would be my saviour at this time. Thus on 12 November:

> *"I rang Nora. She is from the Commonwealth funded carers group. They offer crisis type help for carers. The sleep-over people are from private providers but well sussed out. The cost is met by the Com. Govt I believe. It sounds good and I will make use of it perhaps next week."*

Rosa from St Luke's also rang to say she had contacted the Mater Hospital about day respite for me. Friday 14 November:

> *"Took note that we went to bed by 10pm and then were up at 11.30, 1am, 2.45 and 4.15. I am really tired at the core. Guess the same about Marg. I thus called Nora and have arranged for respite for 12 hours, 8pm to 8am on Wednesday next. Lord only knows how that will go. I also called the Mater Respite Centre."*

The lady from Ozcare who helped with my house work came that same day. She too asked whether there was further care available for me. I found over the many months that once a carer had been with us for a time, she invariably formed an idea of my need which was better than I was capable of doing for myself. Out of my experience I would counsel carers to listen carefully to the advice of others. It is so difficult to be in the midst of things and be able to objectively analyse ones own needs. I am sure it would not be uncommon to 'care to death'.

> "I am fast growing to understand that I can't be a 24 hour carer without support no matter how badly Marg reacts to others."

It was Wednesday, 19 November, when I tried the night respite service. My report of that experiment concluded:

> "Last night was both a failure and a success. Failure in that I got little unbroken sleep. I was anxious as to how Marg would react with Wilma and I could hear every footstep from downstairs. Success in that Marg was OK, went to the toilet only once during the night. Would not let Wilma change her incontinence pants for her though."

I decided that the experiment was not worth following up. On 21 November Marcia from the Mater Respite Centre came to our home:

> "They will start Marg on Thursday next. Seem very competent. Special Commonwealth funded program for carers. Seem to have a good caring philosophy. Am sure Marg was very negative throughout. Only time will tell whether she takes to it or not. It would give me up to 5 hours for myself once a week. Can but try I guess."

I was asked to give the process at least a month's trial. December would be abnormal as the centre closed down over Christmas, but we thought it would be useful to try at least once before then. Naturally I worried myself sick about how Margaret would react to my sending her off to a respite centre. I took it upon myself to try to ensure that she had been adequately toileted before she left home so that she would suffer no embarrassment. It was like getting a young child ready for a first day at school. I packed a large handbag for her. In it I had a change of clothes, extra incontinence pants, a comb, etc. The bus driver, John, arrived at 10.10am on the Thursday:

> "Marg was the only passenger. She looked a little tentative about getting in the bus and more so when I did not stay. Not a good image to carry for the rest of the day. They got back home here at 4.10pm. The other older ladies said farewell. They told me she did well. Had her hands massaged but not her feet."

Next day Marcia rang me to tell me Margaret did grow agitated for a time and wanted to go home. She would not use the toilet but held on for 6 hours until she reached home. Still this looked like a good deal for me and I grew to look forward to having just a few hours for my own needs. It is not easy for the carer not to feel selfish by doing so.

As I have repeatedly said, the two major concerns I faced each day related to sleep, or the lack of it, and faecal incontinence. Of lesser importance in terms of overall stress, but still a cause for concern, was the daily showering routine. From the toileting perspective, my learning's were many though slow.

Though I could coax Margaret to the toilet and have her remain there, the old adage remained – you can lead a horse to water but you can't make the animal drink. My real problem now was just how long to leave Margaret in the toilet without causing her great distress. It made such a huge difference to the quality of any one day if she had a normal bowel movement. My experience indicated to me that we were likely to be successful either just before of immediately after breakfast.

Had I been more aware earlier that faecal incontinence was likely to be a problem, I would have greatly benefited from knowing her normal patterns before the need for assistance arose. I would recommend this to the beginning carer. Take note and take notes so that as time and the disease progresses you have a guide. There is nothing quite like a regular daily routine in so many areas of life for the Alzheimer's sufferer. Unfortunately a normal BM does not necessarily mean that there will not be any further accidents in the day. If they do then occur, they tend to be smaller and thus a lot easier to deal with.

At night the use of incontinence pads was invaluable. By November I had moved to having Margaret use incontinence pull ups made by either Tena or Depend. Margaret found these comfortable and did not seem to mind the change. From a carer's point of view they were so much easier to employ and to change. I would recommend that they be of a kind that can be easily separated down the sides.

Margaret would wake often during the night and sit on the edge of the bed wondering what she would do next. While we were in our queen sized bed I was usually aware of this movement and would accompany her to the toilet. It became more of a problem when I ultimately gave in and put us in single beds, albeit side by side. I did this on 16 November. Sometimes she would now be up and wandering around before I was aware of it. I did have a sensor light set up so she could find her way to and from the toilet. For several years I did not turn off the toilet light.

I found it useful to have adequate shelving in the toilet area itself. There I would store extra incontinence pads, baby wipes and disposable rubber gloves. The large baby wet wipes were far more effective in my experience for assisting an adult after a BM. I also had special washers, towels, soap and barrier creams set out in the nearby bathroom for the cleaning required from faecal incontinence. Napisan was an indispensable tool for the laundry.

Showering was more of a struggle than a real problem. I was pleasantly surprised how well Margaret accepted my help as her need for that grew. She did not accept help from others though. My main concern was the possibility of her slipping. She would lather herself and I would assist only when she had forgotten what to do. Towelling off was a joint exercise which required some sensitive negotiation. It was at such times that tempers could flair. Dressing after her shower did provide a few hurdles. I never had any trouble in the mornings but in the late afternoons she would be a little stroppy. When eventually I installed a hand held shower and placed rubber matting on the floor, much of my concern about her slipping evaporated.

Just as sleep deprivation was the major issue for me, I suspect it will be so for all carers. I can safely say that for three and a half years I never once slept for more than 3 hours without being woken. Many, many a night we would be up 5 or more times and on average we were up 3 to 4 times a night. I never knew what to expect any night either as I noted on 13 October:

> "By late afternoon I was feeling as though I could sleep on a rail. I tried to read but kept nodding off. I had gone into a deep sleep early at night. Woke with a start at 3.15. After a journey to the toilet with Marg she slept only lightly until 5.15 then got up at 6.15. At 3.15 I found Marg could not stand by herself. She kept trying to bend backwards and would lose her balance. OK though later on and through the day."

I was so tired by the end of October that I could not force myself to stay out of bed while Margaret was on the toilet. I wrote of 30 October:

> "Had the air-conditioner on all night. That did not help us have a trouble free night. To bed by 10pm but up at 1.15. Up again at 3.30. Marg was tossing around. Up again at 5.20. I lay down and fell asleep. Left poor Marg in the toilet for 20 minutes."

My modus operandi was to escort Margaret to the toilet, have her seated, then sit on a chair nearby until I was satisfied she was finished. The chair was out of Margaret's line of sight to ensure she had as much privacy as possible.

The fact that we were now in single beds ensured that I was not disturbed by every movement made by Margaret during the night. Of course it did not alleviate the problem arising from her snoring. She would often have mini spasms during the night which would make her bed jump. There was a downside though as I mentioned on 6 November:

> "We had a terrible night. In bed soon after 10 but awake at 1.15 or so. Then Marg was still awake at 2.30. I got very annoyed. She just did not seem to understand it was time to sleep. I put Marg back to bed and then went to the neighbouring bedroom. I

could not sleep I was so upset. Settled as I heard Marg snoring. Woke at 5.30 with Marg up and sitting on the bed beside me."

Eventually I purchased a laser beam operated alarm which I set up by the bedroom door so that I would know when Margaret was out of bed. I later moved the device to a pair of large wooden bookends I owned and would place them at either end of her bed. The beam was set at about shin height. When Margaret sat on the edge of the bed her legs would break the beam and the alarm on my bedside table was activated. If we had a moth in the house or some other flying insect we would have a very broken night's sleep.

To break our normal daily pattern I took Margaret to Burleigh Heads for a short holiday in early December. Our daughter Anne once more accompanied us. It would be the last holiday we would try together. Margaret was very confused. At times she did enjoy our walks and sightseeing. The nights though were just too hard to handle away from our home environment.

Margaret continued to accompany me to mass each weekend. We would enjoy that experience though Margaret by now was no longer even pretending to sing the hymns. I would hold her hand while we went up together to receive communion. Sometimes I would accept the host on her behalf then give it to her. It was necessary for me to do this as all that my lovely wife wanted to do was have a little conversation with the person distributing communion. The normal response on receipt of the host was 'Amen' but Margaret would simply say quietly "Thank you". I thought that was beautiful. If I were God I would have worn a smile from ear to ear.

By the end of 2003 Margaret's eating patterns had begun to change. It was as if she would forget what she was supposed to do. This was especially obvious at breakfast. About halfway through her cereal I could no longer coax her to feed herself. I thus began to feed her once she lost interest in feeding herself. She never fought me over this. Her other meals required that I did a lot of coaxing, but she responded positively. Drinking was not yet a problem as long as her cup had a reasonable handle for her to clasp.

The 'turns' she had in 2002 did not seem to be as obvious. I felt they were now being expressed through remoteness in her general demeanour. She would still say that:

"She does not know what is going on in her head."

Her moodiness was often related to her need for toileting, our Ebixa experiment, lack of interesting daily activities for her, etc. Once in a while she was still capable of ripping a button off her clothes.

Our lives were so totally taken up by the disease and the consequences that I would write on 11 December:

"What a day! I realised it was our 38th wedding anniversary. It really stuck me hard as I put Marg on a bus to take her to the Mater Respite Centre. When I got inside I broke down and sobbed. Every time I think of it I want to cry again."

I followed that up as the year wound down on Christmas Day:

"Anne was our sole guest for lunch. It turned out very nicely. At one stage Marg, with eyes full of tears, told us how happy she was to be with us. I cried, so too did Anne. Margaret continued to have a conversation with Eliza in a picture....Cried a lot today as I looked at Marg and thought about what could have been."

Chapter 7

2004

A Hard Day's Night

As the new year dawned I could not have imagined how traumatic it would become. There were new and developing issues to face while the day to day problems already with us intensified rather than abated. Tiredness from broken sleep dogged us:

> "We were up at midnight first after being in bed by 9.30 for Marg 10.30 for self. Then we were up at 1am, 1.30am and 2.30am as well as 5.30am. I do drop off to sleep but not too deeply. There are times when I sit and wait for 10 – 15 minutes just in case a BM is imminent. I know that is part of the problem usually. At least it gives us a free day later."

As I mention with respect to 2003, I needed a way to detect when Margaret got herself out of bed. I did try an infra-red system as that cost me only $59 compared to the $149 for a laser beam. The infra-red system was a failure for us which is why I turned to the use of the laser beam. Nevertheless, I did have a problem even with this device. When the beam was broken an alarm was triggered but only if I remembered to turn it on before I fell asleep. If I did not remember to do that an incontinence issue would result.

During January I experienced just how important it was for there to be as little change as possible in the personnel allocated to work with Margaret. I recognise that it is often difficult for agencies to allocate staff, but I would suggest that the Alzheimer client must relate to the same person if at all possible. On 6 January our usual carer from St Luke's was replaced by another carer. While they were out having a coffee, I received a call from the carer to say that Margaret refused to get back into the car for her. With much coaxing she eventually did do so thank God. Both the carer and I reported this incident to the agency and we were pleased to welcome back Rosalie. As it was in 2003 so now too did Margaret's demeanour always darken on their return from a successful morning's outing.

Respite recommenced at the Mater on 22 January. Margaret was picked up about 10.30am and dropped off between 3.30 and 4pm. I would take her hand and walk with her down to the bus and ensure she was seated and strapped in. In my mind's eye I can still visualise her eyes staring at me as the bus drove off. Those eyes had the look of one who was being abandoned to a fate worse than death.

> "Marg looked so lonely and deserted as she drove off in the bus. I came inside and wept. I just can't get over how our lives have changed."

We continued to take our walks through the park and around the neighbouring streets. We went to mass weekly though Margaret would at times be so tired, dare I say bored, she would fall asleep during the sermon.

> "I even wonder why we try so hard to get to mass in this weather. It strikes me more so when I watch Marg having absolutely no idea what to do with the host. I tried to say our prayers with her last night. That was a shock too. She did not join in, just said over and over 'that was good'."

Nightmares plagued Margaret at this time. She would wake me by making the strangest guttural noises as if she were terrified. I would wake her and hold her in my arms until she settled again.

On 21 January another part of Margaret's pre-Alzheimer life ended. I rang the electoral office and they forwarded me a form to be signed by our family doctor. Her life as a voter was effectively finished. I found that sad because she had been one who had always taken a keen interest in the political scene.

It was now the case that there was seldom a time when I did not feel overwhelmed by a deep sense of utter tiredness.

> *"What a day! We had a horror night. If I can remember we were up just after 1am then 2.45, 3.15, 5 or so then 6.30. Marg has been spaced out most of the day. She told me she was tired and she felt strange in the head. Perhaps this is yet another dip down in the cycle of life she now faces. I feel tears rise up every time I really look at her, something I would never have done before. Her poor middle toe is black and blue. I hope it is only a bruise. Those toes have no bend in them so it must hurt to walk. Does she complain? No. Do I? Yes."*

It is common to find in my diary notations such as that for 8 February:

> *"We had a rough night. Up 5 times and I must admit I have been like a bear with a sore head at the end of the day. I try not to get angry but it wells up from my toes and blasts into my head. I wish it were different but it is not. Only hope I don't take it out on Margaret. She does not need that with everything else she suffers."*

At another point in this same month, after witnessing her often daily distress, I wrote:

> *"I felt so sorry for her. It is just so removed from herself as she was. I could cry at the injustice of the situation so fine a person finds herself in. I guess I never would have thought in my wildest dreams that this is how we would wind up. I am certainly finding out how poor I am at giving rather than being on the receiving side. I really wonder what Marg feels, how she sees me, whether she sees me as a good person helping her or someone to be feared because I get so angry at times."*

I began to be more aware how short was Margaret's concentration span, particularly in a setting away from home. While grocery shopping I would often have to leave the trolley to gather her in, take her by the hand and lead her back to the trolley. It did make shopping that much more difficult, but I sensed that she still liked the outing. It had been for so much of her life one of her daily chores. Actually, Margaret appreciated going out somewhere every day. That could simply entail a walk in the park with a stop at one of the park benches to listen to the birds.

Margaret's agitation was expressed in a number of different ways. I have mentioned the pulling off of buttons which went on for several months. She now began to rub the legs of her trousers. I purchased a little battery operated pilling cutter to smooth them out for her each day. The rubbing also left her trousers stained. Each night I would simply spot clean them. For what it is worth I had a little atomiser spray of water and some rough cotton cloths which were invaluable in lifting the stains from the trousers for me. I did not find this job onerous at all. Strangely I would get a buzz out of ensuring that Margaret's clothes were neat and tidy for the next day. She had always been meticulous in her dress.

Margaret's shoulder continued to give her some pain. When I assisted her with dressing in the mornings, I would do simple exercises with her to keep the shoulder loose and in use. She would at times give me one of her 'what are you up to' looks, but generally she did not mind as long as the exercises were gentle. I found a product called Perskindol was useful. It had a liniment smell about it and I would massage it into her shoulders and back. I was never too sure whether it was the product that worked or just the daily massage - perhaps both.

I was very much appreciative of the outside assistance I was receiving regularly. I took an opportunity to visit the Mater Respite Centre on 26 February. Margaret and I drove there that day. I was informed that Margaret had settled in quite well. She was not distressed when I left though she was glad to see me when I arrived to take her home at 3.30pm.

On Tuesday mornings Rosalie continued to take Margaret out for a couple of hours. They would generally have a good time together. There was always a little resistance to begin with.

It continued to be the case that Margaret's face would suggest she would rather be anywhere but in the company of her carer by the time they returned home. Rosa would take no offence at that. It was I who felt embarrassed knowing that that was not how Margaret would behave in normal circumstances.

On 9 February I had a run in with Ozcare. I regret that now. At the stage I was at I would have taken on the world for even the smallest matter that I felt would adversely affect our daily life. Our disagreement focused on the type of assistance I was receiving with housework. The particular array of assistance was bound by government regulations associated with the funding provided. Margaret was expected to assist with the housework undertaken. Margaret's inability to help the carer with the work meant that this particular program could not continue. I was a little upset by that and also the way in which it was first conveyed to me. I also thought that there would have been a better understanding of the effect that Alzheimer's had on Margaret's competencies as her disease progressed. My patience was stretched too far when it was suggested that I may be better off seeking private assistance for the type of help I required rather than any Government funded program. I regret that I hung up in a rage.

Ozcare followed up with me in a few days. I had worked in an environment for many years in which government money was the base for many programs. I well understood the restrictions that government regulations could place on the use of such allocations. I had by now become more rational thank God. My head ruled my emotions and I agreed that the specific program was not appropriate for us. It ceased, but Ozcare determined they would seek an alternative for us.

On 18 February the supervisor of our regional Ozcare office visited our home:

> *"She was a delightful lady. She has convinced me that I need to look to have Marg's name down at Aged Care facilities. You don't need to accept an offer and not to do so does not automatically drop you off any lists. Also we are in line for a Community Package when it comes available. Also I need to seriously consider some time out for myself of a couple of days at least."*

My learning from all this was that it is extremely important to ensure the carer fully understands the program on offer and the need to assess its operation regularly as circumstances do change; and in our case they changed rapidly. In the busyness of the carer's life that can be missed. It is also instructive to have those in charge of various agencies actually visit the place of residence to see first hand the realities facing the sufferer and the carer.

Ozcare, I believe, now moved heaven and earth to have us receive a Community Package. I feel very strongly that such assistance is essential if Governments are fair dinkum about helping to elongate the at home care process. There are too few of these packages. Once the number available has been allocated you find yourself in a queue waiting for one of those ahead to move on or die so you may access one. In the light of our circumstances, we remained on the existing package until the new one commenced.

Meantime I had a breakthrough with MASS regarding the incontinence aids. They phoned on 20 February:

> *"Apologised for being so tardy in meeting my needs. Will send a couple of samples by Monday then, when I ring, she will order the special pants for us."*

They did arrive on the Wednesday. On 2 March I was able to place my 6 months' order. Though it could take weeks to fill the order, it was a godsend in terms of cost saving and convenience. I needed a storage place for the boxes when they arrived. If the supply ran out before the end of the 6 month supply period, I found it quite easy to ring the suppliers directly for more aids. Payment for the extra supply was made directly to the supplier. The local Ozcare supervisor visited home again on 2 March:

> *"A day towards change. Rep from Ozcare came at 9.15. Megan was with me. Rep went through the process and documentation for the Commonwealth Care Package. Agreed that for the time being best help for me is housework and some cooking. Also respite care at 2 hours per week on Tuesdays will continue. Can use that program for more such respite including emergency need, overnights and long weekends, etc. The CCP will cost me $76 per fortnight at this time."*

It took a couple of weeks for matters to be resolved, but St Luke's would no longer be providing us with care. I will always be thankful for their service and the personnel who met our needs so well. In truth, I am thankful for the assistance we gained from all agencies throughout our journey with Alzheimer's and particularly the thoroughly professional way all carers treated me and Margaret.

I was now spoiled. The new package allowed for the making of a few meals for us each week. I would freeze them for use in the days to follow. Having pre-cooked frozen meals was a tremendous help. I would never knock back an offer from anyone willing to prepare us a meal.

I commenced the process of visiting nursing homes and then applying for a placement for Margaret. My daughter Megan was usually with me through this emotionally draining time. I hated every moment of it as I thought I was being so disloyal to my darling Margaret. I felt this way even though I knew it was inevitable that I could not look after her in the long term with the resources at my disposal.

In time we visited more than 10 facilities and put in an application to some 14 or so. The quality and range of nursing care facilities was mind blowing. Nearness to our home was a consideration in the selection process, but more so than anything else was the ability of a home to best meet Margaret's needs as we perceived them.

Our first visit to a local home had been a bit of an emotional shock. The facility had been constructed over 50 years earlier and it was tired looking. As with many such places they were planning to rebuild when and if money was made available. We applied on the hope that the rebuilding would have taken place by the time Margaret needed to enter. It reminded me a lot of the state of private schools prior to governments pouring capital money into them. Perhaps we need a Nursing Home Commission to mirror the School's Commission of the 1960s and 70s. The plight of these homes is largely hidden. Each of us possibly will find ourselves competing for the limited places available in the years ahead. We do need to begin to raise our voices because the reality is that the squeaky wheel does get the most oil, especially in the political arena.

Our second visit to another home on our list towards the end of the month was somewhat different. The facility was most attractive, but:

> *"What depressed me was the age structure of the people in care in the dementia unit. They looked so old and feeble. Terrible though the thought is, I hope God is merciful enough to take Marg to Him before the need for such intensive care. While she has slipped a lot over the years she is a long way I suspect from those we saw today."*

Life naturally goes on around you while on this journey. Of great joy was welcoming our second grandson, Sean Joseph, on 18 March. I could not but take great delight in witnessing the love in Margaret's eyes as she held and stroked so gently the new addition to our growing family circle.

Margaret experienced another change on 12 March:

> *"We had a hair appointment at 9.30. I suggested to Mary that we forego the colour process. Mary razor cut her hair. It is very short and rather grey. I think it will take time to adjust to. She looks so different. Marg seemed upset at first as it is her image friend she sees as changed."*

Hiding things was something Margaret did regularly, and regularly I would get cross with her for doing so. Even her food would go missing if I was not paying sufficient attention.

Sleep deprivation haunted us always as I comment on 29 March:

> *"What a night. I can't recall all the times we were up, but having hit the pillow at 10pm Marg was up at 12.35, 1.30, 2.15, 3.30, 4.35, 5.10 and 6.22am. To say I feel buggared is to state the obvious. I lost it at one stage last night and the anger rose up in me. I eventually punched myself in the arm just to do something. Stupid? Yes, but it stopped me from manhandling Marg."*

Some experiences would lift my spirits and, for a time, make all the hardships seem worthwhile.

> *"I had a wonderful experience this morning which brings tears every time I think about it. We had had yet another broken night and before breakfast I was taking Marg to the toilet once again. I hold her hand while we go. Suddenly she came close to me, put her arm tightly around me and with her head on my chest said, 'I really love you'. I could not believe it. Later in the bedroom she gave me again quite a genuine hug. I was over the moon. I can't remember when I last had any overt sign of affection from Marg."*

April arrived and Margaret continued to go to the respite centre each Thursday. I always had a little coaxing to do. I noticed it made quite a deal of difference to Margaret's mood when one of the female staff accompanied John at pick up and delivery. It was also helpful if someone else was in the bus when it arrived. Margaret was by nature very introverted, so she was going to be wary of new faces. At the centre she would most often at least eat her sandwiches. She refused to use the toilet initially until she grew to trust Marcia. One of the staff:

> *"Told me Marg was rather anxious in the afternoon. I think as winter comes on that will be the case earlier in the afternoons and also, I am sure, it is partly due to a need to go to the toilet."*

I would remain home during the four hours that I received help each Friday with housekeeping and cooking. I would keep Margaret company. It was the two hours of a Tuesday during which Margaret went out with her carer that I had time for my needs. Her carer was Janine who used to help during the aborted housekeeping program I mentioned above. Margaret felt comfortable with her and:

> *"Janine tells me she is beginning to see the type of person Margaret used to be and is. Says what a beautiful and gentle person she must have been."*

As the weather was kind to us at this time of the year, we continued to go for our daily walk. We would go at a time that I thought best suited Margaret. Often that would be after lunch rather than in the morning. Margaret would talk non stop while we were out, though the 'words' made no sense to me. I would try to answer and hoped that my response was the correct one. We were still going through her 'fruit salad' conversation phase. It was a little difficult to know whether she was actually talking to me or just to herself. She continued at home of course to talk for hours with her image.

Though Margaret loved being with her children and her grandchildren, she would grow very distressed when noise levels rose. I did note that she was noticeably more at ease with her world and everything in it in the mornings compared to the afternoons. On 17 April we had visited Maree and her children when:

"Marg, full of smiles, said to me, 'Isn't it good to be here!'"

I took Margaret to our family dentist on 30 April. He invited me to stay with her as he examined her teeth. I expected this would be her last formal visit to the dentist.

"I was proud of Marg. She was anxious but did what was asked of her. No holes and needed only a clean etc. She seemed very glad to be outside though."

Margaret's 'turns' continued. Sometimes she would look very pale in the early morning as I dressed her. I thought at times she would faint. I would sit her down for a time. At other times she would dry reach, then she would settle and the colour would return to her face after a little breakfast. During these episodes I saw my role as trying to help her remain calm until they passed.

On a less serious note, Margaret could wander around the house without making a noise. On 25 April I had put her to bed and then returned to the downstairs area to watch a little TV. I watched for a while, switched it off and stood up. Margaret was standing right behind my chair. I had not heard her and I almost collapsed in fright.

Earlier in the month I was, as usual, trying to do too many things at once around tea time. I would set out our night time tablets for us to have before the meal.

> "I took some then realised they were Marg's. Panicked. On Mike's advice rang 131126. They suggested I would be OK and should take my own tablets."

Though I felt a little off in the stomach overnight, there were no adverse side effects. I had treated myself for Alzheimer's and rheumatoid arthritis.

Attending mass was becoming more and more difficult for us. We persisted because of its importance in both of our lives. I am pleased we did so. Religious belief, hope and love were totally integrated into our lives even in this, our hardest journey.

> "Marg was on a high at times today. Responds to cheer and being part of the conversation. I wondered tonight whether in Marg I have a window into the goodness of God. She forgets, forgives so often. There seems to be no residual hard feelings no matter how much I fail in my serving her needs."

Some of our regular parishioners, after witnessing my efforts to look after Margaret, congratulated me. Such words were always welcome though I knew they did not see me when I was not all that good in the caring role. It is unfortunate that we do not appear to have retained a culture in our present day church of providing personalised practical assistance, other than via the specifically allocated institutions.

At a personal level I found that this period of my life presented me with significant challenges to my faith. I wrote on 18 April:

> "We went to mass at Coorparoo at 9am. I find myself at mass often, but wondering deep down, why? I have some answers, but guess it has something to do with pain in the world and some doubt about the depth of my faith. Can but stick in there, pray and hope this aridness of soul will pass, and I will find myself in a beautiful oasis in my desert."

With the help of my daughter, Megan, we contacted more aged care facilities. Most required an appointment to visit though some had set aside specific days in the month for look and see visits. We did get to visit a number during April and May. Our family doctor completed two separate detailed medical forms for us. Formal applications generally required such documentation so I would simply photocopy these and attach them. Nursing Homes did not mind that the form was from another facility. Our ACAT forms arrived on 10 May. Once photocopied, I had all the documentation necessary to make formal applications.

Sometimes in my diary I would be reflective rather than just outline events. At the beginning of May I wrote:

> *"As I write I feel sick to my soul. I have always wanted to continue to treat Marg as an equal partner, my other self so to speak. Tonight I got so upset about her wiping her hands on her good trousers that I lost it and treated her like a naughty child. God help me! As if she would deliberately do anything 'wrong'. She cannot do any thing 'deliberately'. Makes a mockery of the mass we both just attended. I keep asking for help, for strength, for the virtues to care well, and I keep failing. Sometimes I think for Marg's sake it would be best for her to be in an institution. Yet she always forgives me. That is one faculty she still seems to have – to forgive. That has always been part of her nature anyway. She will sit high at the table of the Lord later on, can't see us being close together though."*

I highlight Margaret's willingness to forgive. It was so large a feature of our journey. I note on 12 May:

> *"I thought last night how I must always remind myself that caring for Marg is caring for God's daughter, temple of the Holy Spirit. Whenever I help her, she says simply, 'Thank you, thank you love.' How beautiful, how simple, how apt. God always forgives as does Marg."*

Once in a while I would be given an insight into her ability to see humour and to show understanding:

> "She amazes me sometimes. Saw a very heavy lady on TV at lunch time and she said to me, 'Isn't she fat!'"

I never knew when the appropriate connections would be made in her brain. When she was out with her carer on 11 May they were outside having a cup of coffee under a tree. A bird did its business on the carer. Margaret laughed whole heartedly as did Janine.

About this time I began to take note of what I called 'spasms' that Margaret was having. They were most noticeable in her legs and their frequency was increasing. It is only as I write this description of our journey with Alzheimer's that I can make a connection with her earlier 'turns'. The spasms were so strong that at times I thought that her legs would go from under her. Accompanying them was a new phenomenon. I record on 22 May:

> "I noticed Marg had a lean to her left during the day as if she could not stand straight."

This lean would last for several days. The lean became more pronounced the longer Margaret sat, so I would prop her up when seated. I also employed massage and some gentle exercise. Often the lean would right itself almost overnight, but then it would again reappear in a few days, only now set in the opposite direction. The more pronounced the lean, the more difficult was it for Margaret to go for a walk with me. Her balance was affected. It was obviously very uncomfortable for her. I took Margaret to the doctor. She had no obvious muscular problems and her blood pressure was normal. He did inform me though that:

> "Some Alzheimer sufferers also have Parkinsonian signs or again it may be a reaction to her drugs."

The leaning did worry me and it continued to do so for many months. My own observation was that she had begun to be less mobile during the day and she was spending long periods of the day just sitting. In some of our lounge type chairs there was not the lateral support that she may have needed.

I hated the thought of Margaret ever being in pain. Her inability to use language made it difficult for her to tell me if she was in pain and, if so, where. I began to learn that my best guide was to note her body language. It made me wonder how Alzheimer sufferers ever coped with operations and any necessary hospitalization. As the month of May came to a close I reflected:

> "Some days are worse than others, on the emotional side at least. Could be a culmination of utter tiredness I guess. Today I find myself crying at the drop of a hat. I can't talk about Marg even to myself without the emotions getting the better of me. I know how deeply I have always loved Marg, yet this is not the same person – very little communication etc. I get annoyed at having to be on call all the time, yet I look in her eyes and there is a call – please stay with me, keep me safe, thank you for what you do. She always was a saint in my eyes, she remains so. How hard it is to see her nose run with her cold and she not aware enough to wipe it. She is totally dependant on me and I am so poor at providing her all the support she needs."

As I have said, Margaret's lean to the left or the right remained a problem. It took a different direction on 2 June.

> "I thought it would do Marg good to go for a walk to Annerley Junction with me to get a loaf of bread. On the way home Marg began to walk slightly bent over at the waist. By the time we got home the bend was quite pronounced. It was as if she could not stop moving for fear of falling. She leaned against me and was rather sweaty. Her eyes showed some concern too. Michael rang after we got upstairs which Marg negotiated on her feet and hands. Again she lay against me until I could set her down. I have been watching her closely for the rest of the day. Could be her drugs, could be middle ear, and could be onset of Parkinson's I believe."

To add to the drama of that day Margaret slipped and fell in the shower. Thank God the only outcome was a nasty bruise. I spent the next few days looking for and buying suitable rubber matting for the floor of the shower. It needed to be soft under her feet as well as lending itself to being easily cleaned. That she had slipped greatly affected Margaret's confidence getting into and out of the shower recess.

I planned to buy a suitable shower seat. It was difficult to adequately clean Margaret after being soiled. A shower chair would have been very useful. Unfortunately none that I could find allowed sufficient room in our shower recess for the person to be seated. Eventually I had a wooden slatted platform made to fit into the shower tray. It meant that Margaret did not have to step into it. It was now at the one level. While a little hard on the feet it worked well. I still remained concerned that Margaret could be seriously hurt if she were to have one of her 'spasms' while in the shower. Thank God that happened only the one time during which she cracked her head against the glass.

Margaret's 'spasms' though infrequent were of major concern. Their violence increased quickly as noted on 30 July:

> *"When I was dressing her, always very difficult because she just stands and is very lethargic, she had one of her spasms while I was reaching down for her slippers. She fell on her backside and hit the back of her head on the ironing board legs."*

When a 'spasm' would occur, it was as if for a brief moment Margaret had no muscular control, and would drop like a stone. Usually she would steady herself before hitting the floor. This would normally happen as we walked to or from the toilet at night, but not only then. Afterwards, Margaret would complain of her head feeling strange.

> *"Can never get to understand what that means. Tells me she is not in pain at least."*

Margaret's Thursdays at the Mater Respite Centre continued. I had my hands full as the time approached to talk her into getting on the bus. She hated the idea that I was not going to be going with her. There was a kind older lady who was often on the bus when it arrived. Beryl would help settle Margaret and sit beside her. As they talked I thought, what a lovely act of kindness that is.

During June and July Janine, who was usually assigned to caring for Margaret on Tuesdays, was away on vacation. We were allocated a couple of different carers during this time and it was interesting to watch Margaret's reaction to the changes. Consistency is certainly a necessity for the Alzheimer sufferer. I was pleased to have Jan return, but as she was now seen by Margaret as a third change there were more problems than existed before her vacation.

When life seems to be just one sleepless night after the other, followed by days dealing with all that faces the carer of a loved one deep into Alzheimer's disease, it is hard to remember the few special moments. It is such moments that now jump out of the page at me as I re-read my diaries. On 10 June:

> "Marg always says thanks to me when I look after her. Last night she leaned over and kissed me on the forehead and said, 'thanks'. I could have cried. I was so touched. Love to know what goes on in her mind."

I then record 10 days later:

> "I had a marvellous experience this morning. We had had a good night's sleep - best in many, many months. In bed by 10pm, up at 1.50am and 5.45am then slept in until 7.50am. Marg was very alert in her eyes though she collapsed backwards on to the toilet seat at one stage. I had just finished dressing her and putting on her shoes when she said to me, 'I know you love me. I love you too.' The latter she said with her hands on my face. It was all that I could do to stop from crying. Main sign of affection from Marg in a very long time - years I suspect."

My Margaret continued to enjoy outings. We were part of the local coffee set. Unfortunately our public outings were not always a joy for her. On 28 June we were out shopping with our youngest daughter, Anne, and sat down for a coffee.

> "Marg seemed very agitated and when Anne asked her to drink up she almost began to cry. I have not seen Marg cry for a couple of years. Almost thought she could no longer do so. She

> said to us in a quivering voice, 'Everyone is looking at me.' Felt so bad. May have been her seat faced the glass to outside."

She would feel like this on a number of other occasions. Still I was pleased to see that she never quite lost her sense of fun. She had had one of her short hair cuts. I found it much easier to care for, but:

> "When we got home Marg looked in the mirror and said to her 'friend' she sees there, 'You look like a man' and then laughed."

Lack of sufficient sleep was the hallmark for the month of July. Margaret was no longer sitting up at the side of her bed when she awoke. This meant that her feet did not activate the laser beam alarm to wake me. I had now lost control of our nightly toileting routine. However the human body is truly amazing. In a short time I trained myself to sleep so lightly that I would be aware when Margaret woke during most nights.

I began to notice that Margaret did not initiate conversation with me. I was not sure initially if this was the result of the deepening of the disease, or the lack of restful sleep we both experienced. However, when I would have a conversation with any of the carers, Margaret would grow very agitated and her face would spell out her annoyance. I needed to be sensitive to this.

I would from time to time try to look at our journey through Margaret's eyes. I should have done this more often as I tried on 22 July:

> "Thought today how hard it must be for Marg. Tried to be in her shoes. Sometimes she squeezes my hand in such a way I believe she is saying thanks, or asking to be looked after. I can imagine she must be saying to herself, Vince I can't tell you how embarrassed I am for soiling myself, I don't do it on purpose, I hate having you to clean me, please remember me as I was and you will know how I feel, please look after me, I am totally reliant upon you. If only I could meet her every need without anger."

I am ashamed to admit that, more often than not, my reflections were of the 'poor me' kind as on 27 July:

"There are some times when I sit down to write that my heart is so heavy. I can understand that saying now. I am so dog tired. Could hardly motivate myself to get tea or go for a walk this afternoon. On top of that I got so filthy on poor Marg because she would not wash herself properly. The more irate I grow, the more she becomes almost unable to do anything. It is surely fear. At a time when she is simply seeking security, love and someone to take care of her, she has this totally wild individual shouting at her. I can only guess how that makes her feel. Then I feel so bad about myself and the human excuses seem so frail. Once again I have fallen, once again I need my God to lift me up and get me going again. Perhaps in my heart I feel a great need to get away just for a time, more than a few hours. Then I feel I am being selfish. I ask myself, can Marg get away from her situation - no."

I was desperate to find an answer to incontinence during July and August in particular. I tried to take note of any sequence especially as to the time of day. I figured I was trying to solve a biological problem and just needed to find the right key. I again rang the Commonwealth Continence Hotline and had a useful discussion with one of the nurses. Out of that conversation I began to control the quantity and type of fruit we were including in our diet. It was a period of trial and error; mostly of error I am afraid. Life was very difficult for us both.

It was about this time that I began to suffer badly from a type of eczema. My hands would become red raw with little skin on some of my fingers. It especially was painful on the right hand which I used most often. I did have my hands in water many times during the day and, though I had disposable rubber gloves on hand, I just could not get used to wearing them. I did not feel in control of my actions.

This was not the time I would have wanted to contract a bout of the flu. Nevertheless I got a severe bout which stayed with me for over two weeks. The carer gets no respite from the daily grind and lack of sleep even when ill. I hoped and prayed that Margaret would escape it. She did not, but in her case it was more a severe head cold than a chest infection. However, poor girl could not even blow her own nose. She did not know what to do or how to do it. I had to be ever watchful to ensure her nose was wiped as and when it was required. To help her gain a good night's sleep I used a nasal spray and rubbed good old Vicks on her chest. It did seem to work in the main.

During this period I had assistance from an occupational therapist through DAART. An outcome was the provision of a hand rail support for Margaret's use when getting off the toilet. Unfortunately it was never used. Margaret could not figure out how to use it. She was at a stage in the disease that to learn new activities was not possible. Even if she figured out what to do on one occasion, she would have to re-learn it on the very next occasion.

My daughters offered to sleep over once in a while to give me some night time relief. I was not aware of just how worried all three were about my general health and well being. Those who really love and care for you can often provide you with an objective assessment of your needs. If I take a line through my role as carer, I found the carer was the worst judge quite frankly.

I may not have been as aware as I should have been about my own health, but I was very aware of my shortcomings as instanced on 6 August:

> *"I get so tired from the long days and short nights, the constant non-communication, the irrational behaviour, the seeming lack of thanks for all that you do. None of that is however other than a feeble excuse for my lack of charity – genuine charity – seeing God in Margaret, serving God through serving her, etc. Giving without looking for anything in return is the hardest part of Christian giving."*

Margaret's spasms were becoming ever more obvious and worrying. I wrote on 13 August:

> *"When we were up at 2am Marg had a series of mini collapses walking back to bed. One was so bad she actually landed on the floor. Hell of a job to lift her up. Worried me, and from the look in her eyes worried her."*

We once more visited our family doctor. Her blood pressure was normal for her. That was checked as her medications could have caused a change in her blood pressure leading to the collapses. It was determined that we stop her normal blood pressure medication for a week or two to see if that helped. By 27 August her blood pressure was low, so she recommenced her medication. In my heart of hearts I did not believe the collapses were associated with blood pressure. I admit though that, only with hindsight, I could make a link from her earlier 'turns' to these episodes, and the neurologist's advice that epilepsy may be part of the disease.

Daily life was further complicated by the return of Margaret's lean to the right or left. On our doctor's advice I tried Vallium in the hope of relieving the muscle spasms. I was also urged to use some massage to relax the muscles. Unfortunately I could not get Margaret to lie down so that I could do the massaging effectively. Though it was difficult, I did try while she was seated, but with minimal results. The best time for me to massage her back was just after Margaret had had a shower. That became part of our daily routine.

The Vallium did work when we first used it. It also had the effect of giving Margaret a deeper, more relaxed sleep. I was concerned that Margaret may become addicted to them, so I used the Vallium very sparingly. I had been advised that at this stage of Margaret's disease it would have made little long term difference to her. Perhaps I should have listened to that advice.

I mentioned earlier that Margaret would at times bend forward from the waist. She spent literally hours each day leaning over a bed, a chair, the sofa, tidying her possessions – pillows, teddy, small blanket, etc. I thought that this was partly the cause of the bending forward so I would try to have her sit down throughout the day. She would often let out a sigh of relief as she sat. It was as if she may well have wanted to sit, but could not think how it was to be done.

By the middle of September Margaret was showing signs of a deepening of her vagueness in the mornings, usually until about 9.30am. Its effect was obvious at breakfast. With my initial encouragement she would start to feed herself, but soon she would appear to lose all interest. While this had happened intermittently earlier, it was now a daily occurrence. No amount of encouragement would move her to re-start feeding herself.

To ensure she ate sufficient I would feed her. As she had done before, Margaret accepted that quite calmly and would finish her meal. Other meal times were not a major issue. Cleaning her teeth of a morning was also affected by this vagueness.

> *"I did however get very cross when Marg could not/would not clean her own teeth. This is happening in the mornings, not so at night. I think my frustration is that I see it as yet another skill she is losing. Hate that. Must try not to make her suffer because of my frustration."*

There was a change of carer for Margaret's outings of a Tuesday from 14 September. Margaret had bonded really well with Jan for many months as she had done previously with Rosalie. I was concerned about this change, though I would find I need not have been so concerned.

> *"New Ozcare person Di arrived at 9.40 this morning. She is tall and has a vibrant air about her. She is infectious and that showed in Marg who took to her from the outset. We talked for 15 minutes about what happens, traps to avoid, etc. then off they went for two hours."*

Margaret would now almost look forward to her outings, but by the next week, as I had come to expect:

> *"Marg was in good form until they began the journey home, then as often happens she changed. Was not accepting of help and would not say goodbye. I get embarrassed by such behaviour yet I know I should not. It is the disease."*

We were now receiving assistance from two carers having the same Christian name. The woman who came on Fridays for four hours to do housework and some cooking was also called Di. Thursday respite continued with my ongoing struggle to get Margaret to board the bus. If Beryl was there she would relax a little.

Intellectually I began to process the very real possibility of Margaret being placed in a nursing home. I was trying to calculate how long I could reasonably continue to care for Margaret at home. We had a family get together on 5 September and Anne stayed to help me with the final clean up. I discussed the possibility of a nursing home with Anne. We sat together and cried at the thought.

I tried never to lose sight of Margaret's and my decision of years earlier, when first told of the disease, to enjoy life as far as possible. For now this involved at least our daily outings. She loved to visit the girls. Such visits had to be limited to no longer than about an hour though. Margaret enjoyed our ventures to the shops and our morning cup of coffee while out. There was no drama as long as I either sat directly in her line of sight or right beside her to help her eat the sweet cake I would always buy for her.

When October rolled around, I could not but be concerned about Margaret's continuing to lean sideways. I noticed in showering her that her stomach looked a little bloated. This was strange for one who had been so slim and trim all her life. A visit to our family doctor found no abnormalities other than her muscle tone had largely gone. He suggested that this:

> *"Could be helping her back to spasm. Suggested some exercises, but I cannot get her to follow any directions. He again told me that Marg had deteriorated very rapidly and it will not be long before I need to institutionalise her for both our sakes. I kind of know that, but do not want it to be so."*

I wrote more applications to nursing homes and tried to visit them. Ozcare could provide someone to sit with Margaret on the occasions when no one from the family circle was available. I received our first offer of a placement for Margaret on 7 October. I thanked the facility but said I was not ready for such a move.

Incontinence continued to be a major problem during October. The now normal situation was exacerbated by Margaret suffering a three day bout of diarrhoea. When showering was necessary for cleaning purposes in the middle of the night it was traumatic for Margaret. She looked so confused and wondered what it was all about. Lack of sleep continued to take its toll also. I noted on 12 October:

> "At one stage I put Marg on the toilet then lay down but fell asleep. I woke 40 minutes later to rush out to rescue my poor dear."

Night was a real rollercoaster of sleeplessness followed at times by a reasonable rest for us. I set down as an example what I wrote on 30 October

> "I don't recall a night as bad as last night. Marg seemed to actually enjoy the movie 'True Women'. We went to bed by 10.30 but her mind seemed to be active. Spoke to herself in the dark. We got up at 11, 11.30, 12 & 12.30 then about every hour. She would sit up and put her legs out breaking the laser beam so waking me. 9 times in all during the night. I have been very tired today as I am sure she is. At the end of the day I have little or no tolerance and believe I am a danger to Marg. Want to belt her, but I don't. No fun for her though."

Then on the next day:

> "Boy was I thankful for a good night's sleep. We were both so tired last night we were in bed and asleep by 9.30 I would guess. Up to toilet at say 3am then back to sleep until 6.45. Still feel tired but Oh so much better."

I had by this stage ceased giving Margaret a Vallium tablet at night as she seemed to sleep in the same pattern with or without them. Also, while they did assist her back muscle spasms to begin with, they appeared to me now to be having little or no effect. Massaging and the use of Perskindol were my best aides to fight her propensity to lean.

Margaret's loss of muscle control or 'spasms', which present usually of a morning, were of more concern to me now. I would record on 20 October:

> "Marg began the day giving me a few heart aches. She had a number of her seizure like incidents where her muscles seem to not function for a split second. Was worse than ever before this morning."

Sometimes she would have similar attacks even while lying on the bed.

> *"We were in bed early. Marg woke first at 11pm. We then woke just after 3am and again at 6.30. For me that is a good night. Really needed the four hours in one hit. Marg wet but nothing else thank God. Still jumpy in the morning. At 3.30am I lay beside her stroking her hair to get her to sleep. The involuntary jumping of her limbs is really disturbing for me."*

Early in November I once again tried to see if Margaret would like to watch a movie on television at night. She did always like to sit quietly with me before bed. We sat up on 2 November:

> *"Watched a movie called 'Veronica Guerin' last night. Marg seemed to like it. Got upset when she was killed. She was very mentally active when we went to bed and began the getting up every hour bit. I gave her a sleeping tablet. First for many months."*

I decided after this episode to ensure that our viewing be of less violent shows. I also decided that we would no longer watch full length movies on TV before bed.

I found myself explaining to Diane, in front of Margaret, what I had planned to do while she was out for an hour and a half with Margaret.

> *"Marg was strange going with Di. I am not sure if she misunderstood my saying I had to go somewhere else, but she got in the car and sat there crying."*

That night I experienced how Margaret at times understood what I and others were saying in her presence. I had assumed that the inability to appropriately converse with us meant also that she did not fully understand what was being said. I don't think that necessarily follows. After a series of incontinence issues:

> *"I got mad with her unfortunately. Calmed down and knelt down beside her to say our prayers. Began this again yesterday. She*

does get most of the 'Hail Mary'. She looked at me and said quite clearly, 'I want to stay here'. I told her I would look after her as long as I could. I apologised for losing my temper. She reached up and gently touched my hair and said, 'I love you'. I cried. Find it hard to accept such love after I have been so mean."

Faecal incontinence was a great cross for us both. I needed help, but found it hard to obtain. Rightly or wrongly I would sometimes gain the impression that my being a male was certainly no help. I remember how it cut me when a female nurse told me that they had many things to deal with and incontinence was not a priority for them. I felt like screaming down the phone that it was one hell of a priority for us and had been so for a long time. I rang three Government sponsored bodies seeking help and, as in the past, found that help first from the Coorparoo Community Centre. I required assistance in trying to access new pads for both day and night wear as well as in trying to work out a bowel regime and diet. The help was finally gained, but only after I badgered a number of people.

During this year I had to watch my Margaret undergo a change in her own behaviours while using the toilet during the day. The behaviours never showed themselves at night. As she sat on the toilet, Margaret began to talk to someone. I could never make out who it was she was addressing. In a few weeks this talking became quite loud and angry. It was as if she were chiding someone. She would reach out and take hold of the hand towel and give it a good dressing down.

Still later on she would hit whoever it was she was angry at or frustrated with. She would strike the wall nearest to her and later still began to strike her own legs. I would get so distressed that I would have to intervene and ask her to stop. At these times she would look at me with a look of wonder and remoteness. Her thighs would at times be quite red from her slapping them. What made it harder to hear and witness this sort of behaviour was that I knew my Margaret as one so gentle and calm of nature. I could not help but wonder what our neighbours might think because, from outside, it sounded as if she were under attack. Once in a while I would deliberately wander around the backyard hoping to be seen there, so that people would know I was not bashing up my poor wife.

I could never judge when this might happen. It was not associated with every visit to the toilet. I found it necessary to explain her behaviour to regular visitors. Like all of these aberrant behaviours it would eventually abate and then disappear. I often wondered whether it was her only way of expressing her frustration and anger at not being able to control her own toileting needs. I guess I will never know.

Lack of sleep among other things made for huge mood swings in me. To add to them I contracted yet another heavy head cold and sinusitis. Nevertheless, Margaret's needs were always my prime concern:

> "Did take Marg out this morning for a coffee at Fairfield. She needs to get out each day. I am just not feeling up to doing too much at the moment. Very hard to tend to another when you are sick yourself."

I found it difficult to maintain a proper balanced perspective when Margaret would get very agitated at my talking to the female carers while they were in our home.

> "I note again how Marg seems to get agitated when I am talking to other women in particular."

Interestingly, such agitation was not evident if it were our daughters or my sisters I was talking to. When we went out for a meal, I would have to assist Marg with her eating.

> "Marg is not comfortable eating out and I have to feed her. Still I don't get embarrassed any more though I sense at times she might."

Margaret was beginning to look for bed by 8 to 8.30 at night. She may not always stay in bed for long. During the day she was now sitting for longer and longer periods in the lounge chairs. She ceased chatting to the cushions or any item she happened to take with her. She continued to enjoy her outings with Di on Tuesdays and, though slow to get onto the bus, the same seemed to be the case for respite of a Thursday.

Margaret was capable of moments of clarity as noted on 9 December.

> *"Up early to begin the day. Marg was really spaced out even at breakfast. I perhaps get an insight into how she will ultimately become. Even now I think these periods are growing more frequent and lasting longer. In the midst of them she sometimes says things that are memorable. Like this morning when she suddenly seemed to recognise my presence and said, 'I really love you' and tears filled her eyes. Within a short time that moment was lost but I can at least still remember."*

The issue now causing me the greatest concern was her mini collapses. Fear of the unknown I am sure helped that to be so. Of an incident on 18 November I have this to say:

> *"After breakfast I thought I would take Margaret for a walk. She seemed OK, but up near Mrs Diamond's house she just collapsed like a pack of cards. I could see it happen as if in slow motion. Picked her up. She was not hurt as far as I could tell. Left me ashen whatever about herself."*

I got Margaret home that morning and as the day progressed she grew stronger. These collapses would, as I mentioned before, often happen at night on the way to or from the toilet. I usually was holding her hand so more often than not she did not actually fall to the floor. However on 10 December:

> *"I am not sure what happened after breakfast, but I heard Marg plop on the kitchen floor. Luckily she had not broken anything at this stage but I am concerned. I can't see that she tripped. She was sleepy even throughout breakfast. She has been twitching more lately. I just think it is one of those muscle collapses. She needed to be hugged when I stood her up. Says she did not know what was happening but looked very concerned."*

That night she again appeared to lose her balance. I needed from that point to be more careful of her every movement.

As this year is brought to a close I will cite two quotes from my diary. The slightly humorous one from 30 December:

> "Gave Marg some Xmas cake at morning tea. She loved it. Had 2 pieces. Then she picked up one quarter of the cake and took a bite. I had to laugh."

The more serious reflection is of the last day of 2004:

> "Last day of an eventful year. The night was broken and Marg had a bad morning. The little turns she has seemed to come in waves. Even while lying in bed she was racked with spasms. At one stage she totally collapsed in the bathroom while I was washing her face. I get really scared at these times. She did not want to eat or drink at breakfast. Later when I told her to get up and move she left the kitchen but in a couple of minutes was back. She hugged me and did not want to let go. She stroked my back and talked on in her garbled way. She too was scared. I have not wanted to leave her out of my sight for long periods today. At morning tea we sat and talked – exchanged noises – for 15 minutes. She had tears in her eyes at times."

Notwithstanding the fact that I had visited a fair number of nursing homes and received two offers of placement which I refused, I was not to know that this would be our final full year at home together. I was determined to keep Margaret with me no matter what happened, but in the end the price being asked was too great for both of us.

Chapter 8

2005

Final Months at Home

I began the year trying to be positive. I was not as aware as others were how much the years of caring had taken toll on me. My positive outlook did not last too long unfortunately.

> *"New Year is a time to rethink, to set goals, etc. I am mindful that 40 years ago this December coming Marg agreed to be my wife. What a lot has happened, and no one would have guessed we would be dealing with early onset Alzheimer's. On my wedding day I knew so well Marg was God's gift to me. She always expressed her desire to be first and foremost my best friend. Took a long time for me to understand the significance of that – but she knew. In our darkest years – now – I am trying to recreate that sense of Marg as my greatest gift in life. She is even now God's gift to me and what I do with that gift may well determine my eternal position. If that is my goal, and then to live by that goal, I am going to need tremendous help – from God, from family, from friends. I hope I am as successful as I wish to be."*

The carer is on call 24 hours each day with just a little break at night for some sleep, all the time watching the deepening of this dreadful disease in the one so loved.

> "Marg has been rather withdrawn, talks a lot to herself or imaginary others. She seems to have lost a lot of interest in everything really. I could cry as I watch her so deteriorate. I have even given up the fight to have her clean her own teeth. It is too frustrating to try to force the issue. Bought a soft brush so I don't hurt her gums."

Margaret began sitting for even longer periods during the day. She had difficulty getting herself out of the lounge chairs once she got settled there. Her method of seating herself was to hover above the seat and then plop down. She sometimes would land on the wooden arm of the chair and then have a very nasty bruise for days. Bruising was a problem. She would often walk into things that were projecting. It was particularly the case when exiting the car in the garage. I noticed on one or two occasions that she had bruising on her face, normally around the chin area. Lord only knows how she got these as she never did complain or cry out, at least not that I heard. On 18 January:

> "I noticed Marg was dark around the left eye. The bruise from the chin area seemed to have travelled up to the eye area as well. She does not complain, nor did she when it happened."

Margaret did love to sing. I guess I can carry a note, but don't class myself as a singer. However, in the sanctity of our home, I would sit with Margaret of a morning and sing hymns. She no longer joined in,

> "But she would just listen and tell me I was doing OK."

The spasms continued most noticeably in the mornings. She developed another quirk in her behaviour during this month.

> "Notice Marg walking around the house calling for Megan more and more. I just assume it is 'Megan' she is looking for. I find it rather tragic. She certainly sits a lot more - often in Maree's bedroom - talking to herself in the mirror doors."

I was never sure that it was actually Megan, her second

daughter, for whom she was searching. For a time this behaviour seemed all consuming for my dear wife, as I suggest on 23 January:

> *"Marg has been walking around the house calling out for 'Megan' a lot today. In fact can be having a conversation with her and others while I am sitting with her, as if I am not there. She will sometimes be startled by my presence and say hello to me as if I have just arrived."*

People may and did think I had rocks in my head when I decided to have a couple of days on the coast with Margaret from 10 January. Anne, God bless her, came with us. I had assumed that we would never take a break like this after our last experience. Perhaps I am a slow learner. No matter how careful I was about choosing the right place for us to rent there were difficulties. The most significant was that the shower was over the bath tub. Margaret had difficulty stepping into the bath and even more difficulty stepping out of it. Poor dear could hardly lift her leg high enough. She was scared of slipping. Never again I thought, but I treasure the memory and wrote on 12 January:

> *"Anne has been great these three days. She cooks without complaint. We cannot be a lot of fun to be around. I guess it helps me re-realise how great are the gifts Marg and I brought into the world. I know how much Marg loved them all. Bit of a burden to have to carry it for us both. Guess I left a lot of that to her in the past."*

The more Margaret became totally dependent on others, the more I would delight in seeing the way our grandchildren accepted their grandmother. We now had four grandchildren under the age of five – Emer, Tom and Sean (Maree's children), and Eliza (Megan's daughter). In their innocence they had a way of accepting what was, even if they did not understand. They would simply react to her need, as I noted on 15 January:

> *"There is a lovely little image from this morning with little Tom holding his grandmother's hand helping her up and down the back stairs. I wont forget that image."*

Tom was not yet three years old.

Margaret continued her Tuesday outings with Di. The day would begin well for as long as I did not have too long a conversation with Di. During their time out Margaret's moods could vary dramatically. On 25 January:

> *"Marg went out with Di this morning. When Marg is receptive she is so child like. She touches Diane's face and hair and tries to talk with her. When they return though it is a different Marg. I sometimes feel embarrassed yet I know I should not. This is not a controlled action."*

Thursdays were set aside for respite at the Mater which started up again on 20 January.

As with the year past the two areas of major concern for me revolved around showering and incontinence. Showering was a daily 5pm fixture. There were other times when incontinence meant that another shower was required. It became a particularly difficult task when, as often happened, a shower was necessary around 2 or 3am. When Margaret's poor backside had been scalded or chaffed that would exacerbate any problems. Whatever the difficulties, I knew that my main task was to ensure Margaret was clean and comfortable.

As I tried at least to ensure that motions were firm, dietary change was always on the cards. That at least aided in the cleaning process. I seemed to have very little success throughout the month of January. To have some control over this issue of incontinence was a pivotal concern for me. I write on 6 January after cleaning my love for the third time in the day:

> *"I am finding this very hard to cope with. As I consider every thing, it would send me over the edge as far as institutionalizing her."*

I found myself both angry and frustrated at my unrealistic expectations of Margaret.

> *"Marg cannot help being as she is. She does not deliberately try to annoy me. She genuinely cannot understand and hence*

> *follow even simple directions, yet I keep expecting her to act naturally, at least as a child. The fault rests with me not her."*

What I would do in the near future, and what I should have had the sense to do earlier, was to chart Margaret's bowel movements. My hope in doing so was to reduce the guessing and try to bring regularity to her toileting. It was to prove to be an instructive exercise and one I certainly would recommend to any carer who has a similar problem to cope with. As I advised once before, start this charting even before there appears to be any real need. When I was successful in the toileting regime as I was in the first 3-4 days of February, it is hard to express in writing the level of relief that created.

Most days I felt as though I could go to sleep on the floor. Being so tired so often made me less appreciative of the pleasant times that were had.

> *"Marg went out with Di today. Marg was in a great mood and did not mind the time out at all. I think she talked all the time."*

On 4 February I indicate how good are the times without incontinence.

> *"Slept reasonably. No bowel problems again. Must remember the good with the bad, when the bad returns."*

Every six or so weeks we continued to travel to Stones Corner for Margaret's regular haircut.

> *"Marg had her hair cut today by Mary. She is a lovely lady who seems to delight in looking after Marg. She would not let me pay as it was for Marg's birthday."*

If my memory is accurate, Mary gave Margaret a complementary bottle of shampoo and conditioner for her birthday. Some people are indeed very special in our journey and it is a great privilege to meet with them along the way.

Though Margaret's birthday is 7 February, we had the family get-together on the day before as it was a Sunday. We went to mass. Margaret was beautiful the way she said thanks to the person giving out communion. After Mass we had a BBQ.

> *"Marg seemed to sense she was the centre of attention. She got quite emotional after we sang happy birthday to her and gave her a present. I was too emotional to read the card to her."*

I wrote on 7 February:

> *"Margaret's birthday today. She turns 66. I find it hard to believe it is now five years since our neurologist gave us the devastating news of Marg's condition. She had a fairly good night and again BM not a problem for me or her. I could get used to this of course."*

I knew that life had to change and change it did. By 12 February we were back to being up some six times during the night. We were both dog tired. Sometimes Margaret would get herself out of bed. At other times I would find her asleep on the toilet and I would wonder how it was she did not fall off.

On 14 February I had an episode that I experienced several times over the years. I thought that lack of sleep was the major cause.

> *"Another broken night. Went to bed by 9.45 but up at 10, 12.15, 2, 4.15, and 5.30. I was beset by a spinning head early in the morning. Only way to stop the room spinning was to prop my head up on a pillow. Been a while since this has happened and it worries me. Last time could find no cause. Perhaps lack of sleep over 48 hours does it."*

Our family doctor found my blood pressure was normal. I began to wonder whether lack of sleep also had something to do with Margaret having spasms because on this day:

> *"Marg had a collapse this morning while I was putting out the washing. I thought I heard something but did not investigate. Found her still sitting on the floor of the dining room. Seems to be no bones broken or pain. A real worry though."*

Final Months at Home

Up to this point I had been nearby when such events happened. I now had another matter to add to my daily concerns for her safety and well being.

Life is full of surprises about the things that we see as important. For instance it was important to me that I began to notice a pattern from my graphs with respect to Margaret's regular bowel movements. Between 2 and 3pm each day was a time to be watchful. This at least gave me a clue about timing. However my level of tolerance was in the decline as I note on 19 February:

> "This time I gave her a shower. She pushes me away physically when I try to wipe her and instead of remaining calm I get annoyed. I am sorry for that. The disease is getting worse and I find it difficult to put up with the drivel she speaks all day. At other times she is silent."

This is the first time I can recall expressing myself like that about my beautiful wife. It frightened me that I felt the way I did. The topsy-turvy state of my own thoughts and emotions showed themselves on 20 February:

> "I find myself almost in tears as I look at Marg these days. It is so cruel that she cannot converse. I just wonder what life is for her. She cannot tell me of course but I wonder at the frustration, fear, loneliness of it all. I hope God does not let her linger into complete oblivion."

Then the very next day:

> "I had upset Megan unfortunately. Told her that I felt perhaps to die would not be a bad idea for me. I was down this morning and I really should learn to keep my mouth shut. They all have enough on their plates without me adding to it."

Still, life went on with its little moments of exquisite joy. On 24 February:

> "Marg out to the Mater today. Seemed to be OK about it. Gave me a kiss on the chest when she got home."

We continued to attend mass. Margaret was growing more anxious about the time it took – almost an hour. Receipt of communion was also even more confusing for her. On 6 March for example:

> *"Marg would not accept communion from lady, just wanted to talk to her. I took the host for her and she ate it. May not be long before we give that great gift up too. Can't see that is in God's plan."*

Grocery shopping was now far from joy filled. Margaret would grow very anxious in the store and talk incessantly. I think the fact it was crowded, noisy, and with bright lights did not help. But it was not only in the store that her behaviour was like this. We had a new phase in the disease.

> *"Walks quickly around the house telling 'whoever' off, or that is how it sounds to me."*

It was not limited to in the house either.

> *"Went to the chemist after lunch and walked around the block. She talks non-stop and anxious talk too."*

She did so love shopping though for as long as we did not stay beyond an hour. It did not surprise me that she loved going shopping. I was always amazed, throughout out married life, how often she could be there for so long a time and come home with next to nothing. I would often plan our shopping excursions so that we could meet up with someone like Megan and little Eliza for coffee. To have Margaret try on clothes before buying was no longer an option. I would now buy clothes, bring them home to try on her, and more likely than not have to return some for another size. I got quite proficient at shopping for her needs and knowing where to look, particularly for petite sizes.

I had thought that Margaret would never go to the dentist again after her last visit. I decided to try one more time. We went to our long term family dentist on 11 March:

> "I went in with her. She was a little scared. Doctor was good. Spoke to her as he would a child. Checked, cleaned and used fluoride as best he could. No real damage to teeth he could see."

I should have warned the dentist that Margaret may not be able to rinse when asked. A mouth full of liquid was always swallowed; although I had two rather humorous experiences involving rinsing. I am not sure how humorous I thought they were at the time.

The first happened one evening after I had finished cleaning Margaret's teeth for her. I would try to get her to rinse and spit out rather than to swallow. From the bathroom we proceeded to the kitchen where Margaret would have her three Melatonin tablets before going to bed. I would give her a drink of water after she had chewed them sufficiently. Chewing these tablets was never a problem. On one particular night I gave her the water; she swilled it around in her mouth then spat it on the floor. The second incident occurred on 27 March.

> "Gave Marg a drink of water before bed, she swilled it then spat it out on kitchen table."

I quickly learned to let a little time pass between teeth cleaning and final bedtime drink. I enjoy recording experiences which give one great hope for the world of our 'younger' generation. I had called in to a personal training establishment nearby to get some assistance with my at home training regime. It was agreed that one of their personal trainers would call in on me at home to assess my exercise program and make any necessary adjustments. I knew there would be a cost involved. He arrived on 2 March:

> "I went through my routine with him. He offered some suggestions but said largely I was doing everything he would advise. When I asked to pay him he would take nothing. Said I had enough to care for and he had done nothing for me."

I was astonished that a complete stranger could be so compassionate and kind. It meant a lot to me and I do hope that fortune has smiled on that young man.

For some time now Margaret was wearing pull up incontinence pants 24 hours a day. The summer months were very hot even though I had installed ducted air conditioning in our home to try to make life a little more bearable for Margaret in particular. I should have been far more aware of the heat generated by wearing such protection all day. My awareness was raised when Margaret began scratching herself, at times very violently. Sometimes she would scratch until she would bleed. Leaving the air conditioner run all day and using talcum powder seemed to alleviate this problem.

I would hate to have to put a value on which month of any year was worse than others, but I notice that almost every page of my diary for March suggests 'a bad night'. On 3 March:

> "Another bad night in that I could not get Marg to have a BM. Maybe 7 lots of soiling in the past 36 hours was enough."

And the next day:

> "Some nights are worse than others. Last night was bad in that we were up 6 times and from 5am to 6.30 I don't think Marg stopped talking, if you can call her words talking."

From 5 March I began again to keep a daily chart of Margaret's bowel movements. As I said earlier, this was a tool I could/should have used years ago. Lack of sleep associated with incontinence took its toll physically:

> "I have had a head 'ache' all day. It is the type of head I associate with lack of sleep. I even had to lie down for 15 minutes in the afternoon because I just feel exhausted. Funny thing is I have done nothing physical all day though. Sign of a need for a break I am sure."

When we had long periods of broken sleep, Margaret would also react by being 'away with the fairies'. To be balanced, I should note that not every night was a total wipe out, though at times it seemed that way. My note of 15 March says:

"One of our better nights. I think how the night goes is the hallmark for the carer. We were up only three times. Marg had a BM at 4am. We had been out to the toilet an hour earlier but somehow I knew she must go again at 4 thank God. She slept in today until 7.15. Even so she has been in a strange mood all day .... Has been talkative but with anxiety in her voice."

Looking back through my diary I recognise that Margaret would often suffer from spasms after a sleepless night or being woken by me from a deep sleep. 18 March :

"Glad the night is over. Got Marg up at 11.45pm. I thought she was awake. She began to have fairly violent spasms while I was dressing her after a toilet break. Had two more on the way back to bed, then they continued fairly violently while in bed. I stayed beside her stroking her hair. She settled after 10 minutes. We were up a further 4 times before breakfast."

My dear Margaret continued to suffer from her sideways leaning and lack of balance, particularly after walking. In the light of all that had happened so far in 2005, I can better understand the tone of my reflection of 19 March.

"I am finding the caring role very, very difficult of late. I seem to get so angry over what is very little on reflection. For example when I had to clean Marg's teeth and she will not let me gain proper access, then swallows the rinsing water instead of spitting out. I feel so terrible after my reactions and Lord only knows how Marg feels. She cannot tell me to buggar off, she is totally defenceless, and she has a disease which is causing all this in the first place. There is no excuse for other than care, love and security for her at this stage. I will have to consider whether she can get that better somewhere other than being with me. But I really don't believe that in my heart of hearts."

So tired was I , so worried were my children growing about my physical and emotional health, that, at long last, I began to look into the possibility of taking a couple of days off for myself. My daughters assured me that they would be with their mother most of the time I would be away. We hoped that this would assist Margaret to accept a professional carer looking after her. Thus on 23 March:

> *"Rang Commonwealth Carers. They later called back. They had not had a case where daughters may be around. Costs about $25 an hour. Same person for whole time. Cost met by Government but ask if I can pay something. May be all the girls have to do is be on call rather than stay. I guess I am going to have to hope it all works out."*

I had a major internal battle in my heart and mind over this proposal. It was as if I were about to abandon my best friend even though I knew it was for only 2 – 3 days. My disposition was not helped by events of 29 March.

> *"Had two conversations with Marilyn of Com. Carers today. I have offered to pay $50 a day for their help. Had been far too generous in my previous thinking as I am offering food, lodging etc. for the carer who will come. Her name is Sheila. Can now try to get used to having 2 days away. Marg got very teary after my telephone conversation. She must understand more than I think. She said, 'Are you going away?'. I was shocked. Has been close to me all day since."*

I had often suspected that Margaret comprehended much more than I would have reasonably suspected of one deep into Alzheimer's. I reminded myself again to always talk to her as if it were the case she could understand, though could not articulate an appropriate verbal response. I would do so also if I were talking about her in her presence. With the help of Commonwealth Carers, I made plans to take a short break at the end of April. April would confirm how broken sleep appeared to make Margaret more susceptible to her spasms. It further underscored that they were more prevalent when I woke her out of a deep sleep. On 1 April:

> *"We were up twice. One occasion I must have woken her out of a sleep. She slumped to the floor on the way back to bed. Takes all my strength to get her up."*

During the days following such episodes I would note:

> *"Marg has been really out of it all day. Almost like she has fallen a cog in this disease's progression. She is getting very shaky on the steps too. Almost fell today."*

I came to understand that my darling Margaret's depth perception was being destroyed by the disease. When we were at the top of the stairs she was not able to discern each step. It quite possibly looked to her as if I were asking her to take a step into a large hole. The dark nature of the carpet on the internal stairs in our home would not have helped her at this time either. I began to understand why she was so hesitant in negotiating sets of stairs. Later in the month, 20 April to be exact, I again write:

> *"I note again how difficult it is when I try to get Marg up when I don't realise she is still asleep. It is at this time she has her collapses and is very non-cooperative."*

I recorded on that day the physical impact on me of her collapses.

> *"My right hip muscles aching badly by end of day. Must have hurt them when caught Marg in a fall last night. Hope it is better by tomorrow."*

I did usually manage to catch Margaret before she reached the floor. On this occasion she was about to get back into bed. As she collapsed I caught her and in the one motion hoisted her, or flung her, onto the bed. Stupid now I think of it. I could have done my back in rather badly. The following night Margaret had a number of minor collapses. At such times she would buckle at the knees but right herself before a total collapse. In the busyness of our daily living, I had forgotten that I had been told that some Alzheimer sufferers do have epileptic episodes. In fact the neurologist had indicated to us years earlier that Margaret's last EEG's had indicated that such episodes were a distinct possibility. He indicated they could be controlled by appropriate medication.

I grew to expect the episodes following sleeplessness. Strangely they could occur, albeit less frequently, even after a good night's sleep, as I note on 29 April:

> "The night was long. Marg slept soundly, but though I went to the other bedroom I still could not sleep. Marg had a BM in the morning thank God. She actually slept until 8am today. Even then did not want to get up. When she did she collapsed after her wash. Fell so heavily I thought for a moment she may have broken something. I got her up but she continued to spasm for a long time after. Had to sit her to clothe her for the first time."

This was the morning of the day I had arranged to take my two days away from home.

The lean that Margaret had developed early in April was not now as obvious. No amount of massaging had worked so I tried Vallium for the first time in quite a while. Though it left Margaret acting more remote, it did work to a degree.

Of growing concern was Margaret's lack of mobility and inability to carry out simple instructions, like to lie down on the bed at night. I wrote on 23 April:

> "Not too bad a night. During the night I have great difficulty getting Marg back into bed. She seems not to know what to do with her feet. I just wonder how Megan will go next weekend while I am away."

It was also the reality that our walks had to be kept short.

> "Took Marg for a 30 minute walk after lunch. Felt bad about it. It was too far for her. Will have to keep it shorter in future. Poor love really struggled. She has a noticeable lean still. Just can't get it to right itself at this stage."

Added to the above was my observation on the 25 April:

> "Note that it is becoming harder to get Marg to stand after she has been seated for a time. Also she seems unable to figure out how to lie down at night after a visit to the toilet. Need to lift her

feet onto the bed then spin her around before she lies down."

Thank God Margaret was never a very heavy person. Just to finish off the emerging picture, I wrote on the same day:

"I hate bath time. I almost always do my block. Marg does not cooperate. I think she is even more scared than ever about balance etc. I really don't know how much longer I can look after her as I now do. Feel really bad even writing that but in another 6 months it could be very difficult."

I should have mentioned that Margaret had a very heavy head cold during the first part of the month. We had had a flu shot on 5 April and that may have made things worse. It lasted a good 10 days. Try as I might I could not teach Margaret to blow her nose or even to wipe it. I made sure that the tissues we had were very soft as her nose grew ever tenderer. The stuffed nasal passages did not help either. The woman who claimed she never snored could now drive me to another room without much effort.

We continued to go to mass during April. Margaret would talk to me throughout the service. What she said was incomprehensible, nor did she speak in a whisper. I was pleased that people in their charity did not stare at us or make us feel uncomfortable. I was uncomfortable enough as it was. On 10 April we went to have a coffee with Anne after the mass. Margaret grew very distressed as we waited for 20 minutes for the coffee to be served.

"Marg got distressed. Feigned drinking without a cup then poured some on the floor. I try not to get embarrassed though I am aware of all the sideways looks."

Only now do I see this as a strong statement by Margaret of her disapproval of such poor service.

During April as in many months of my records I am made more aware of the tremendous support that I received from our extended family. My two sisters, Helen and Colleen, were often on call should I need an extra pair of hands and someone to sit with Margaret. For her part Margaret seemed to accept them into the house without any real fuss. Other members of the family would assist as their working circumstances would allow.

I received our reissued annual high care assessment from ACAT on 26 April. The assessment is valid for 12 months and if not acted upon it must be renewed annually. Workloads for those doing the assessments were high. The reapplication process needed to begin at least 6 weeks before the end of the current assessment. At the reassessment meeting it was suggested that I may be able to access a new program aimed at helping to keep high care people home longer. It was specifically targeted towards dementia sufferers. To take it up if/when available would mean leaving the care provided by Ozcare. That had its difficulties as I had grown to trust and like the carers who served our needs on Tuesdays and Fridays i.e., the two Diane's. There would be no adverse implications for the day respite at the Mater, whose care and support went beyond simply respite, as I record on 21 April:

> *"I had a call from Mater. They just checking in. Nice of them. Suggest I think of Marg coming twice a week e.g. Monday and Thursday. Said Alzheimer people do not see accurately - steps, doorways, etc. Should consider taking an offer if at place really like."*

When the day arrived for me to begin my few days respite, I could hardly bring myself to go. With Margaret in the capable hands of Sheila and Megan I left, feeling like a traitor.

> *"I was really distressed at leaving them. Marg wanted to get in the car with me. I cried off and on until I got to Nerang. I felt so bad but know I need a little break. Rang Megan. All was well then."*

When I did return from my two days off:

> *"Marg's eyes lit up when she saw I was home. I think she recognised me and certainly wanted to hold my hand."*

Sheila, who had cared for Margaret, said of her experience:

> *"Was surprised to see someone so far gone as Marg is still being*

cared for at home. She worries about the collapsing. Suggests a gerontologist. Also concerned about showering while standing. If falls should get an ambulance to come in case she is hurt."

Sheila's honest assessment of Margaret's condition was a shock for me. Living with Margaret daily, I was blind to what was the reality. It was the type of honesty that was needed to have me gain a more balanced perspective. For a short time after the break I felt on top of things again.

"Am very tired still but feel more at home with my role. Marg gave me a genuine hug after breakfast. She seemed suddenly to note it was me with her."

I did not have long to wait before my new found enthusiasm would be put to the test. By the middle of May I was informed that we were on the waiting list for the new dementia program. I had begun with Megan's help to review all the nursing homes we had contacted to determine how we might best proceed. Together we nutted out an action plan and determined a short list of facilities. The latest ACAT assessment had to be copied and forwarded to all those on our list. We also determined to ensure that we visited all the facilities as yet sight unseen. We then tried to place the homes in an order of priority should offers be made and I felt the time was right to accept an offer. Non-acceptance would not exclude Margaret from the facility, but it did normally mean a long wait until she was considered again. One of the facilities we had contacted in 2004, Nandeebie Centre of Care, rang us to say they would now accept an application from us as their waiting list had been shortened.

I had all sorts of intellectual and emotional problems facing up to what was beginning to look inevitable. When then I refused an offer of a placement from a nursing home, I wrote on 25 May:

"I have found myself crying throughout the day just thinking of what it would mean for Marg more than for myself. Yet I am sure that if she is looked after well it would be best for both of us. Then I wonder if my self interest is getting in the way

> ...*The girls say they will stand beside me whatever decision I make re their mother. Appreciate that greatly ...I think I am becoming more convinced that I should move to having Marg in a home of our choice in the near future. My heart is so heavy just thinking about it. Still we may both have a better life. At least that is my fond hope."*

My two days break at the end of April did not cause the change in my thinking. Rather I was fearful that we may ultimately not retain control over the choice of home for Margaret. That choice could well be taken from us if I fell ill, or if Margaret herself fell too ill for me to continue to effectively care for her at home. Our limited finances would not have allowed me to hire someone privately as a carer. For years I had been trying to do what would normally be done by three people, each working an eight hour shift. I was extremely tired and all I had to look forward to was a further deterioration in our daily circumstances.

Shopping together was a real challenge. Margaret would wander off and I would bring her back only to have her wander off again within a few minutes. She would talk loudly and incessantly such that I was forever asking her to be quiet. We missed mass on a couple of weekends. It was finally time for me to arrange for one of my daughters to stay with Margaret while I went off alone.

> *"I found it very strange not to have Marg with me."*

I still do.

The spasms and collapses continued. On 8 May:

> *"Marg had one of her collapses today. I am very anxious watching for it these days. I was able to ensure she did not fall heavily. During the day she has had spasms. Even while having lunch it was so bad at one stage she involuntarily tossed her roll halfway across the room."*

I gained the impression that these events were growing in severity. By 27 May:

> "Marg had major spasms. She almost collapsed on a few occasions then was very jumpy in bed for at least 20 minutes."

Internally I would panic at these times. Outwardly I would try to remain calm, speak softly to Margaret, lie beside her and hold her gently. She always loved to have me run my fingers through her hair, so I would do that.

Margaret's Tuesday outing with Diane was growing more difficult. I hate to admit it, but my Margaret began to use language that she hardly ever used in her life. In fact she had made up her own 'swear' words to use. I, on the other hand, had no such inhibitions. On 10 May:

> "Marg did not want to get into Diane's car today. She even swore – said 'shit'."

Both Diane and I had a great laugh because this, with 'bloody', was perhaps the extent of Margaret's swear vocabulary. On 24 May:

> "Marg was very reticent to go down the steps. Di tells me she talked anxiously most of the time. Hard to get her in and out of the car. Even says 'shit' at times. Later Marg tried coming down the internal stairs by herself. Tripped but saved herself from a fall."

Then on 31 May:

> "Di had a hard time with Marg. Took 20 minutes to get Marg to leave her seat after coffee. Swore at Di, 'shit', and pushed her away. I could tell Di was upset. I have suggested that the Tuesday be now at home."

These incidents caused me to consider giving up the Tuesday program and having Margaret attend the Mater Respite Centre on both Monday and Thursday. That offer was still on the table.

On a lighter note, we did have two good social experiences. On 15 May we went to a picnic lunch on the Brisbane Corso with my two sisters, Helen and Colleen. Margaret loved the time out. I had as usual to keep an eye to not staying too long. It was especially necessary as the afternoon wore on. Later, on 28 May, we had a simple evening meal with Megan, Ben and little Eliza.

I had often been advised to attend a meeting of carers. I gave in and attended one as the month of May came to a close. The meeting was held at the Mater. I was the only male in the group. It did help me to realise there are others travelling the same road, albeit that each one's journey is unique. Guilt certainly loomed large in their stories when taking time out for themselves. None of the cases exactly mirrored my own situation. While all struggled with dementia sufferers, my Margaret was the only one who could no longer form words in any reasonable fashion. Margaret continued to go to the Mater on Thursdays. It was quite a struggle to coax her onto the bus and, as it would drive away, she would continue to haunt me with the most soulful of looks.

The following six weeks or so were a time when I went through a personal hell. I realised that looking after my loved one was just too difficult for me alone. Guilt is a very powerful force in our lives and I suffered greatly at its hands. It was time to make decisions and then to live by them. In reaching a decision I was driven by one thought only, seek what is best for Margaret. Whatever that ended up as, I would accommodate myself to it. In other words, no decision I made would be based on my convenience. On 1 June I met with Megan:

> "She had contacted a few institutions to arrange visits and/or to say it is now urgent. As she told me my heart sank. What a difference between the head and the heart. I will never be certain about the timing. I just hope this is the right time and we choose best for Marg. She is my other half well and truly and I feel like I have been told I am to lose half of my true self."

How deeply this decision was weighing on me is, I think, illustrated by how I felt spiritually on 5 June:

> "I went to mass but could not get into it. I so missed having Marg with me. I felt abandoned by God and felt that I was too great a sinner to dare to participate. Communion was of little comfort."

I began to feel myself sinking into a state of depression. I was very tired and emotionally fatigued. Sleepless nights were the norm. Incontinence remained a problem, snoring was not helped by Margaret again developing a severe head cold, and now her loud anxious talk would continue into the night. Her lean, particularly to the right side, continued, as too did the frequency of her spasms. On 10 June:

> "Marg slept fairly well. When she got up about 2am though she had a terrible time with spasms. It makes me so anxious. Even when I got her back to bed the spasms continued. She had the shivers and it lasted for about 5 – 10 minutes."

Margaret was good for the rest of that day:

> "Afternoon went slowly. Marg was talkative. If she were not so mobile and 'talkative' at times it may be easier to see her in a home. I just hope she can forgive me when it happens. I love her so much I can't really bear to think of her not being here. When she leaves it will be for good. I cry even as I think of that. What a way for us to end our lived relationship."

I cry even now. I recall that on 14 June I took up an old prayer book I used many years earlier when I was in the seminary. In it was what is called "The Thirty Days Prayer" to be said to the Blessed Virgin Mary, Mother of Jesus. Both Margaret and I had developed a close prayerful relationship with Mary over the years. It is suggested that Mary would respond favourably to your genuine request if you said the prayer thoughtfully and reverently over thirty consecutive days. That night I began to pray that we would be led to a nursing home, no matter where situated, that would meet Margaret's needs now and into the future. My faith tells me that Mary did listen and my prayer was answered as I hope becomes evident. Earlier that day:

> "I sat and talked with Marg for 15 mins. after breakfast. She talked and I responded. Her eyes said everything, her words said nothing. Later I sat with her and sang hymns. She was in a beautiful mood when her carer came."

I had no way of knowing how long it would take for a suitable placement to become available. We had decided to await one from our own short list of facilities even if that were to take several months. Of the offers we had received we were not satisfied with their dementia care facility. On 11 July we revisited one facility that was high on our short list and were given some hope that Margaret was now high on their listing also. At that meeting I was asked point blank:

> *"What would I say if she rang me in the next week or so? I said I would say yes. My head says that but my heart is so heavy at the end of the day. I feel emotionally washed out. Even when I think of Marg in any such environment, or what to pack etc. I weep again. I know I have prayed and asked Mary to guide me, but I find it hard to give in to my faith."*

To say no to an offer could mean having to wait for another 6-12 months. Life went on at home and with it Margaret's collapses. On 3 July:

> *"Early in the morning I put on a loaf of bread. We went to Yeronga Park for a walk. When we were down near the swimming pool Marg fell. We walked back to the car. I noticed she had grazed her hand. There was blood everywhere. I cleaned it up then we called in on Anne. She gave me some plaster for her fingers."*

I thought that I should try to have another short break. I arranged that to occur late in July. My doctor advised taking 2 weeks away not just two days.

Even though we had our short list of homes for Margaret, Megan and I decided we should finish our visits to possible nursing homes we had originally listed even though they were not on our priority list. I rang Centrelink also to gain as much information as I could about the cost involved in a placement for Margaret. I wondered how I would ever make ends meet when I had to fund myself as well as Margaret separately. Finally on 13 July, the last day of my 30 days prayer, we visited Nandeebie Centre of Care at Alexandra Hills some 25 kilometre from our home. I wrote:

> "It was perhaps the nicest place we had been to. Very clean, caring, chapel and chaplain, family style building. Far away though, and long wait for the places available."

Megan and I both knew, when we first walked into Nandeebie, that it was where we wanted Margaret to live. On the drive home I never spoke a word and Megan tells me she was not game to say anything for fear of offending me. We both felt immediately that this was the best place for Margaret, but we felt we had left our run too late. If only we had visited earlier was our common thought. That afternoon we received an offer of a shared room from another facility. I refused as I knew Margaret could never handle a shared room. The very next day my diary opens:

> "As days go in one's life this could be one of those directional days after which one's life will never be the same. I am emotionally drained as I write."

I usually wrote my diary entries on the evening of the day. In the afternoon of 14 July, just one day after our visit, I received a phone call from the manager of Nandeebie.

> "A woman died overnight, a room is available in the dementia specific area and they thought of us. I was both elated and depressed. I rang Megan. She was over the moon."

Once I could get on to the manager, she suggested we mull it over during the weekend and decide before Thursday next.

> "I cry every time I think of Marg being away from me. I believe this is no coincidence. I have to believe Mary is answering my prayer. Why else has a person died and we the first considered."

It sounds so very harsh that one person must die for another to gain a place, but so often that is the simple reality. It is a frightening prospect for the future as the population ages.

Naturally when the new day dawned I wanted to visit the place again and my daughters, Maree and Megan with their children wished to visit also. My sister Helen, God love her, came yet again to sit with Margaret to allow us to go.

> "I must admit I was even more taken with it the second time around. There are only 16 people – all women – and they are at various stages of dementia. They loved having the kids there. There were activities going on all the time....The room will be good with access to the enclosed court area. We will have to hand stitch her name on all her clothes etc. We met the activities person. The physical surrounds are just lovely. I think this will be just the place for Marg – one I am sure she would pick for herself. I will confirm our acceptance on Monday. Will probably need to have furniture in on Tuesday and Marg in on Wednesday....I am emotionally a mess I must admit."

Margaret would have her own en-suited large room which we could set up like her bedroom at home by using her own furniture and photos. Emotions ruled my days. On 16 July:

> "I found myself in tears often today. I guess I can look forward to that often over the next few days. I am sure though this is best for Marg and, if I am honest, best for myself too. I just pray to God to have the strength to get through it all."

While my feelings were raw over the next few days, I gradually moved to acceptance as I suggest in my note of 18 July:

> "I want to cry every time I think of what we are about to do yet somewhere deep inside there is a place of calmness as I know/I hope this is best for Marg as well as for myself."

The following day the furniture was taken to Nandeebie and my daughters helped me to set up Margaret's new room. The room actually looked great. It would become an extension of our home. That is how I saw it and the policy at Nandeebie made that easy to accomplish. The last thing I ever wanted was for her place of residence to resemble a hospital ward.

On 20 July my beautiful wife would enter Nandeebie. She would die there some 15 months later. I cannot do better than to reproduce my diary of this day to indicate something of the event in our journey.

> "Would not want to go through another day like this. Yet I know that somewhere down the track there will be a funeral. I am sickened by the number of farewells associated with this disease.
> Marg slept well. She gave me her beautiful smile of recognition when I woke her for the final morning at home here. Almost 38 years we have lain side by side in this home.
> Maree and Anne were a tower of strength and help to me during the day. Marg talked to me all the way to Nandeebie. I felt she was trying to say it was OK. That was my interpretation. I was emotionally drained at the end of the day trying to control my emotions. Lost it though when I finally said goodbye at 5pm – tea time. I cried as did Megan on the way home. I feel rather empty now like as though part of me is somewhere else. I still love Marg as I have loved no one else.
> The room looks lovely. The paperwork is largely done. She does not like the toilet area. I rang at 8pm. She ate all her tea and had settled well for the night we hope."

One method of caring had now ended and another was to begin. With the day to day activities no longer mine alone to bear, I wanted to reclaim my role as Margaret's loving, caring husband and best friend.

Chapter 9

The Nandeebie Period

I guess there would be those who feel that, having gained a place in a nursing home for their loved one, the role of carer has come to an end. Their loved one is in the care of others and so, in a sense, they are released from their obligation to continue to care. I have seen this often enough to know it is a reality. For me, as for many others, it was simply a new phase in the care journey. In effect I now had a team of helpers to aid me in looking after Margaret. My revised role would allow me to return to that of loving husband. This change came at a price. Perhaps my diary of 21 July makes for a good reference point:

> *"Last night I had my 'Augustine' night. Alone and in the dark I broke down. As I lay looking at the empty bed beside me the emotions were overwhelming, yet I needed to cry silently for Megan's sake in the nearby room. I lay awake for some time thinking of the times I was short with her and how much now I miss her non-talk, her snoring, the stroking of her hair as she went off to sleep. She always wanted me to be her best friend and last night I was so aware that I had lost my best friend – not lost really."*

It seemed an eternity before I could visit her and see for myself how she was coping. From here on until her death I would spend at least 3 – 4 hours each day with her at Nandeebie. Some days I would stay longer. The great benefit of our new situation was that, if I could not get to be with Margaret for any reason on any day, I knew she was being well cared for by dedicated staff.

Initially I tended to visit Margaret after she had finished her lunch. I would take her for a walk around the lovely grounds. I usually had some afternoon tea for us to have as we sat beside the two duck ponds and talked. I did all the talking, Margaret just listened. She enjoyed these outings as much as I did.

Margaret was at least 20 years younger than the vast majority of the ladies in Kanaipa, the dementia secure court. Four residents could sit at the one dining room table and the ladies seemed to like to sit in the same places for their meals. At Margaret's table one of the ladies was 96 years old. She and one of the other ladies adopted Margaret as their 'bubby'. Margaret looked so young to them and they often thought that she was my daughter. The oldest lady, Doreen, would often give me the rounds of the table because they recognised that Margaret was in a worse state than most of them. I was told I should take Margaret to a doctor and have him cure her. Over time I got to know all the ladies in the court and would treat them as if they were part of our extended family. I would, for example, bring in a cheese cake for birthdays if I knew the birthday girl had no family coming to see her.

My experience highlighted the importance of the primary carer being around in the first few weeks on entering a nursing home. Institutional care is of its very nature different to the very personal care provided in the home setting. Of a daytime, for example, there were two carers and a registered nurse to care for the 16 residents in Kanaipa. The work loads are very demanding. I am sure that all nursing homes would wish to be able to have a higher ratio of carers to residents than operates generally today. Funding levels are far too meagre as too are the salaries for those in whose care we place our loved ones.

In her new environment Margaret had no way of advocating for herself. That was to be one of the aspects of my role. I needed to have the courage to speak out for her when it was necessary. Whenever I noticed that the level of care was not quite what I expected for Margaret, I would approach the two women in charge. I had great confidence in their ability and their integrity. I had my first meeting with Annette on 27 July.

> *"Told me Marg has settled in quite well. She is showered every second day and if she is soiled. She is having a bowel movement twice a day – early morning and after lunch. A physio will see Marg soon. Podiatrist also to see Marg. Asked after my own welfare. Often can be a bout of depression. I must be in the throes now. Marg in good form."*

In these first weeks I chose to act as Margaret's personal carer while I was with her. I would toilet her and, if she was soiled while we were out walking, I would bring her back to her room and clean her. I was later advised that I did not have to do this. It was the role of the carers. Still I did not mind in the first few weeks. I suppose it helped me to adjust to our new form of existence. Sometime later I would stop doing these things and simply bring Margaret's need to the attention of the carers. I am sure though that my looking after Margaret was appreciated by those with so many calls on their time.

At the end of July I was settled enough within myself to have three nights away at Noosa. The pattern of broken nights haunted me for many months; indeed it still affects my sleep. Try as I might while away I could not sleep through the night. I was, however, no longer guilt ridden about taking the time for myself. I knew that Margaret was in good hands and that the family would go to see her as often as they could. I returned to see my Margaret after lunch on 1 August:

> *"Called in on Marg. Got the greatest smile of recognition. She almost jumped out of the chair. Has a lean from sitting at an angle. Diane and Leanne told me Marg has settled so well. She will give them a kiss when they wake her. She does look very calm and settled. Even says she likes it. I guess life with me had grown hard on her as well as me. I brought her a caramel slice for afternoon tea ...She also looked deeply into my eyes for 10 seconds once and I felt her reach out to me. I cry just thinking of it."*

When we first arrived with Margaret I had been asked not to take her off campus for a week or two so she would settle into her new environment. I now began to take her out occasionally for a short drive to Capalaba for coffee, or to Cleveland or Wellington Point.

She loved these outings, especially when we would meet up with members of the family including her grandchildren. Margaret particularly loved to walk out along the jetty at Wellington Point. Often we would have a Cornetto ice-cream before we returned to Nandeebie.

I gained the permission of our parish priest to take communion to Margaret once a week. After just two weeks I formed the opinion that Margaret no longer had any idea what was going on so I ceased the practice.

For the first couple of months I took Margaret's good clothes home with me to wash and to iron. The heat of the water legislated to be used at the nursing home would ruin delicate fabrics. Later on I kept a few good clothes at home for use in case Margaret needed to 'dress up' and the rest I left for the laundry to do. All woollens were best cleaned outside the centre. There was a hair salon on site. I arranged for Margaret to have her hair cut about every 6 weeks.

Management asked if I would write a short 'Life of Margaret' to be placed on file for all staff to read. Such a document meant that those interfacing with Margaret would have an idea of her background, likes and dislikes, etc. In this way it was hoped that both carer and Margaret would feel more comfortable with one another. I finished it on 8 August. As well I put together a photo album of her life. If residents were having a bad day, it was often useful to have them sit down with a carer and look through the album.

It was mid August when I felt I could better help Margaret by being present at Kanaipa of a morning rather than during the afternoons. I would arrive about 10am and stay on until after her lunch. She was normally ready for a rest after eating. Margaret needed help with her meals, so it was also of assistance to the carers to have me there to feed her. They appreciated any help given. It also made me feel part of the family to be able to do little things. At times I would set and clear the tables, take the trolley back to the kitchen, even pump up the tyres of the wheelchairs.

I had hoped that Margaret's anxiety and behaviour while being toileted would change in this new environment. I noted on 18 August:

> "She is even wilder now than before on toilet. I could not help but cry while listening to her."

Each resident has a very specific care plan developed to meet their special circumstances. Once prepared the primary carer is asked to read it, discuss any issues including changes they may wish to propose, and then sign off. I did so for Margaret on 23 August and sought to discuss some items therein.

I was interested to learn that shower time for Margaret was causing concern for some staff. It seems she was hard to control and even that she was "hitting her own forehead and crying". I was not surprised because Margaret would only ever allow me to shower her. I am sure she must have found it quite difficult to get used to a number of different people now sharing that responsibility. I noted that there was little or no trouble for some of the carers. I determined that regular meetings to discuss Margaret's progress was a must do activity.

While I had a growing list of issues about Margaret's general care, none was life threatening. My honest assessment was that the standard of care varied with the carers. I had the utmost faith in most, but not all of them. The hard part for me was having the intestinal fortitude to actually state the truth to management as I had experienced it. I worried that there may be some form of retaliation against my defenceless Margaret. Such fears were proven time and time again to be unfounded. That speaks volumes for the professionalism of the administrators and the carers.

I brought Margaret home for a visit on 4 September for father's day. It was an enjoyable day. Megan accompanied me to Nandeebie on the next day to meet with the facility manager and the clinical nurse. We needed to raise some issues concerning particular staff.

> "Had a good meeting over 2 hours with Annette and Robyn at Nandeebie today. I disliked having to name people but, then again, I must advocate for Margaret who cannot advocate for herself. Megan's support was great. Maree, though unwell herself, looked after Eliza while we were away."

I was not yet fully at peace with Margaret being in a nursing home. Though much has already been said before, I wrote on 5 September:

> "I have been rather weepy today. Got no idea why. Yes I do. I just miss my best friend so much. She always said to me, from before our engagement onwards, that she wanted me to be her best friend. I have no doubt she was my best friend and while I miss her as wife, mother to our children, I miss her most as my closest friend who has unstintingly shared the pains and joys of our forty years together. Today more than other days lately, I just feel her absence, her tenderness, her understanding. I would do anything to have her back with me to share in this glorious autumn or winter of our lives, which could have been the pinnacle of our journey together. I just hope and pray she finds it OK that I cannot look after her anymore, and that somewhere inside her she knows how much I truly love her."

On 10 September I recorded a typical morning with Margaret which was joy filled. She loved her daily walk with me and the treat I would bring for her to eat. There was always plenty of food for all residents, but I would delight in bringing them, particularly Margaret, something special. I was feeling more comfortable in raising any issue related to Margaret's level of care, especially if it related to those matters laid out in her care plan. No one ever complained about my doing so. It was rather the fact that I was encouraged to do so, because unless the issues were brought to the attention of those in charge nothing of substance could be done.

Margaret was one of the lucky residents in that she always had visitors. I was with her each day with few exceptions. Maree and family would visit as often as they could manage. Anne made the weekends her time to come and later on would bring her Richard too. Once or twice a week Megan and little Eliza would accompany me to Nandeebie. Eliza, who was just two years old, would take over the place as if it were an extension of her grandparent's home. As time went on the grandchildren would call Nandeebie 'grandma's home'. Margaret loved the attention. She would show her annoyance through the scowl on her face when the other ladies tried to dominate the attention of the children. Life continued to go through its cycle. On 26 September:

> "Got to Nandeebie about 11.45. They were seated for lunch. Marg seemed very agitated. I asked about her bruised hand and elbow. There was no report written about it. I sat with Marg during lunch. She was very angry throughout .... Took her to the toilet. Success. Went for a walk. She was calmer. When I said goodbye she actually kissed me. I can still feel it."

Two days later:

> "Got a bit of a scare with Marg today. Megan and Eliza came down separately as they need to get home early. Marg was still finishing her breakfast when I arrived. I changed her into her walking shoes, but she needed to be toileted before we went out. I noticed she seemed to lose her balance and go backwards. When we walked she wanted to drag herself towards her left side. After we had morning tea at Wellington Point, she almost fell backwards again. Mentioned it to Cath. Thinks it may just be another outcome of the disease. God how I hate it. She will fall a lot if this happens to her. Can't bear to think of that and the consequences."

I follow this up on the next day:

> "The carers told me Marg had fallen yesterday afternoon. I had noticed how badly she is leaning to the left and has lost her sense of balance. I walked with her in the enclosure. She was very unsteady. Annette came with Catherine. They will set up a session with Dr Colquhoun. Suggest it is like Parkinson's disease. May well be a further deterioration with the disease. Will have to use a wheel chair from now on it seems. She may have more falls. I have been crying about it all day."

I had been around the nursing home long enough to know how serious falls can be for the residents. How my Margaret would ever cope with broken limbs and a stint in hospital was beyond my comprehension. Nor was this the only problem. When Megan and I arrived on 30 September Margaret had black gunk all over her teeth and lips. She had obviously picked up something from someone's room and tried to eat it. We hoped it would do her no harm, but it did again show the safeguards I had at home were not possible to the same degree when living with others. She was in good spirits though.

> *"She was very jerky today and still has great trouble with her balance. Can't help but think it is the next stage of this terrible disease."*

As October began Margaret's lack of balance and spasms seemed to intensify. To ensure that I could get help if it was necessary the carers gave me a walkie – talkie when I took Margaret for our walk around the grounds. There was a wide soft belt that was used to help people while walking. I now used one to ensure she did not fall.

It was time for me to purchase Margaret a wheelchair. There were facility provided wheelchairs in the court, but I figured it would be useful for her to have free access to her own. It cost $799, but it did give me great peace of mind when taking her out in the grounds. Her lean to the left created its own problems even in the wheelchair. She needed to be propped up with cushions. The obvious joy on her face when we went out was reason enough for me to continue our daily outings.

On 27 October Doreen turned 97 so I bought a large pavlova for her birthday. She would love to regale me at lunch times with the story of her father as the pilot and lighthouse keeper at Gladstone. She thought I was from that area also. She also loved fishing and would give me hell for not going out fishing more often. I hated fishing to be honest. Her story would be the same every day. I would listen and respond appropriately. In many respects it was like having a verbal history lesson. She would try to help feed Margaret when I was absent and often told me how Margaret would look for me at night.

Some days Margaret was more agitated than others. At such times she did not seem to recognise that I was with her. Thank God such times were balanced by good experiences. On 8 October:

> *"Maree arrived and that animated Marg. She 'talked' a lot to Maree and I sense that Maree's infectious laugh was good for Marg."*

When we entered Nandeebie it was necessary to have a GP attend her. Dr Colquhoun accepted that role for which we were both grateful. Given Margaret's condition he thought that we should try the drug, Risperodone, in an attempt to alleviate her agitation. It was distressing to me to see her agitated each day and it must certainly have been distressing her. There was some evidence that this drug could be of assistance to Alzheimer sufferers although it was normally used in the treatment of schizophrenia. Its immediate effect was to make Margaret calmer. Later it had the effect of leaving Margaret very tired and sleepy most of the day. She was so relaxed that she could often not hold her head up or keep her mouth closed and hence dribbled a lot. Shortly, with the nurses' and the doctor's approval, she was taken off the drug much to my delight. It was kept on tap just in case Margaret had a severe attack of agitation. Margaret was back to her 'normal' though calmer self in no time.

As with all aspects of the deepening of this disease, it was I who had to change too. I had hoped that Margaret would maintain her mobility much longer than she did. I took her around the grounds in her wheelchair. At some point along the way I would get her up out of the chair for a short walk to try to keep some muscle tone. I wrote on 17 October:

> *"After a time she collapsed. She looked pale. Her blood pressure was down. I got the wheel chair to take her back to her room. She got sleepy and was difficult to feed. God how I love her and miss her. She has the most beautiful smile."*

I should have been more aware of the changes to my love, but in the day to day of life I was often blinded to the realities. On 25 October:

> *"At lunch Cath asked if she could talk with me before I left. I always wonder what it could be. Annette arrived and we met. They have concerns about Marg's deterioration. They think the brain stem is now under attack hence the head bending back,*

> *crossing her feet when standing and clasping her hands. I lost it in front of them – my weakness. She will have to be moved by staff in her wheel chair now. I can still take her for walks, though shorter. They feel she will lose her ability to walk sooner rather than later. I was so distressed I cried most of the way to Sunshine Beach. Glad, so glad to be with family tonight."*

Though I did not consciously refer to it then, this showed how fortunate I was to find a placement for Margaret when I did. Most of Margaret's day was now confined to a regency chair. I would wheel her out to lunch in it and after lunch she would be toileted and then settled in the chair for a sleep. I would put on a CD of her favourite type of music to play lowly in the background. She was asleep before I left.

It is amazing the little things you miss. One of the carers, Diane, told me how she loved to wake Margaret in the morning because of the smile she got from her. That used to be mine to receive. As the disease deepened, Margaret's signature was her smile. It was as if nature had given it to her in compensation for the loss of her power to speak coherently.

Margaret and I were 40 years married on 11 December. We had been planning a little get together at our home for immediate family and significant friends. As the month of November progressed, it became obvious that taking Margaret home was not an option. Margaret needed to be in the comfort of her regency chair for most of the day. Thus we shifted to having the event celebrated at Nandeebie on 3 December using caterers. The hall in the grounds was ideal for that.

The senior nursing staff were always sensitive to my needs, God love them. With that in mind Annette organised for me to meet with a counsellor. I had never done that before other than perhaps in a confessional. I found the session very therapeutic and would recommend it as the tension grows during the life of the carer.

On 30 November, three days before our anniversary celebration, I wrote:

> *"Out to be with Marg as usual. She was sleeping in her room. She had been too sleepy for breakfast it seems. Cath tells me they will*

> *feed her early on Saturday. May be best to let her sleep long and take her over at 11am. I showed her the large copy of our wedding photo. She seemed to get very upset – tears in her eyes…..They had a BBQ lunch. Marg ate little but drank OK. She seems to forget to swallow at times. Can sense that will be the next thing to go. This is not the right way to come towards death. Hate it."*

Finally 3 December arrived and the early preparations for our anniversary celebration meant that the day fell neatly into place. Two of Margaret's regular carers, Diane and Rhonda, came. Margaret was beautifully dressed sitting up in her regency chair. She was sleepy at the beginning:

> *"Woke at 12.10, stayed wide awake until the end, did not eat much, Rhonda toileted her for me, food was good as too the drinks."*

Even in the depths of her disease Margaret knew that this was a meaningful event. She seemed not to want the day to end and was delighted to 'talk' to all who were there.

December was so hot that I went looking for and purchased a portable air conditioner for Margaret's room. Her room had the early morning sun on it and, while that was lovely in winter, it made it excessively hot in summer. Though the air conditioner cost $720 it was very noisy and was only moderately successful in so large a room. As well the tray for the evaporation was too small for the amount of water generated in the high humidity. Within a few days I had to acknowledge that I had once more acted on impulse. I had it replaced with a reverse cycle wall mounted air conditioner. That made life for Margaret in her regency chair so much more comfortable.

One of the carers, who later became a nurse, paid me a lovely compliment on 6 December. Nicole gave me an early Christmas present by saying:

> *" 'Vince I hope my husband turns out to be half the man you are. You are a marvellous man'. I was embarrassed and said it was a life long , for better or for worse commitment."*

I mention this not to heap praise on myself as I know how often I failed in the role of carer, but to suggest that you just never know what positive effect your work as carer may be having on others who observe you.

I eventually applied to be a volunteer at Nandeebie. As a volunteer there were things that I could then do to assist the centre when I was visiting. On 11 December, our wedding anniversary date:

> "At lunch Diane placed a cheese cake box in front of us. I thought it may be payback, but it was a cheese cake with a chocolate 40th Anniversary message. They also organised a hot meal for me too. Betty sang the 'Anniversary waltz' for us. I was very touched. Love being with them all."

Why I thought it may be payback was that I had previously left a cheesecake box in the fridge with a note indicating it was for Diane, who loved cake. It was empty. It seemed to alleviate the stress of life in the dementia court to have moments such as this. It certainly helped me. Any little thing out of the ordinary that Margaret did was now an item for my diary as on 14 December;

> "I got her up out of her regency chair. She walked very slowly with me to the dining room. I was so proud of her. She sat there until after her lunch. Looked tired when I was leaving though."

Margaret slept a great deal of the time now. She often fell asleep after her breakfast and would be dead to the world when I arrived to be with her mid-morning. By lunch time she may be fully awake. I found it a struggle to keep Margaret interested in her meal and awake during the lunch period. I did not worry greatly if she did not eat well since there was a plentiful supply of fortified drinks and other supplements for her. She would usually drink well even if she had little interest in eating. I note on 19 December:

> "Marg was asleep. She woke early – had breakfast – then slept. By lunchtime she was still fast asleep – snoring and relaxed. We decided not to force her awake for lunch. Diane told us how lovely it is to wake Marg in the morning, you get a beautiful

smile of recognition and she calls Diane 'mum'. It makes Diane's day. I am at once so pleased, yet another side of me hurts. She used to give me that beautiful smile when at home. I was warned about these things but they still hurt."

Christmas was fast approaching and there were many yuletide activities at Nandeebie. On 21 December I went to be with Margaret for tea rather than lunch. I wheeled her around with me as we went through the 6 courts to sing carols to the residents.

"Marg fell asleep in her chair. Put her to bed. Left at 7.30pm."

Singing was an activity the residents loved. A young man would come fortnightly to play a portable piano and sing for them. Many of the ladies would have their hair set for the occasion. I was amazed how important music was as a therapy throughout the entire facility. Some of the ladies could sing almost any song from the 1930's and 1940's you would mention. Margaret's Christmas gift to me came early. On 23 December:

"Got out to Marg by 10.30. She was wide awake so I got my smile from her today. It makes me feel so good."

For Christmas day I went against all good advice and drove Margaret home to be with the family for a time.

"It was a tiring event – physically and emotionally and I am sure it is the end of yet another phase of our lives. Margaret will never come to this house again yet her spirit is embedded in it. I missed her so very much today even though she was physically here. I lay her on the bed downstairs after lunch and then I broke down. Seeing her there, so frail and so remote, made so many memories well up within me. That was our bedroom for so many good years."

All the family thought the day was well worth it. I drove Margaret back to Nandeebie at 3pm. The next day was my birthday. I went to be with Margaret.

"She had not woken up for breakfast. She was still in bed. Was

so different to see her lie there. She woke soon after I came. I got one of her beautiful early morning smiles. They then showered her, etc. Her poor legs look so emaciated. No walking means she is wasting away…..They had an ice-cream cake for me. We shared it with the residents. Love being there at times. The ladies all have their moments and Diane, Frances and Cath handle it all so well. Boy they give of their time and energy."

The year was coming to an end. Some of the staff were as surprised as I was at the rate of the progression of Margaret's Alzheimer's.

In Kanaipa court there was never a dull moment. Good old Doreen at 97 years of age, after watching me like a hawk (she always did so at meal time) and seeing my frustration with Margaret when she would not eat, took me by the hand and with a twinkle in her eye said,

"Patience is a virtue you know".

Maisie would regale you with stories of her being one of the first nurses in Queensland and driving a T-model Ford throughout North Queensland. Lizzie would wander in and out of others' rooms causing many an altercation. Phyllis, the little bomber, would threaten to blow up anyone who was not on her wave length. She would tell us that she was an expert because of her time making hand grenades during the war. Betty wanted a man, any tall man would do. She loved to sing and had her own version of some tunes that would turn your head. Ruby always wanted to go home because the kids were missing her, while the other Phyllis looked on and just read and re-read the paper. She died before I got her the Yatala pie she always wanted.

There was always lively banter and some practical jokes between myself and the carers. All this added spice and variety to my hours with Margaret in a court which sometimes reminded me of that movie, "One Flew over the Cookoo's Nest". You just had to assist the residents, laugh with them, and sometimes even shed a tear for them.

Margaret's participation came down to saying "I'm sorry" after she sneezed, or ask at table, "What are they saying?" She said little else, though her eyes seemed to take it all in.

Margaret's spasms returned with a vengeance as 2006 opened. She also was looking for more daytime sleep. Often the two went hand in hand. She was losing weight. I had purchased several sets of size 16 trousers for her when she came into Nandeebie. They all had elasticised waists and needed to be of that size to pull up over her incontinence pads. She was now swimming in them. I went out and purchased several size 14 trousers. I kept some at home for a while. She never did wear them. I eventually gave them to one of my sisters when Margaret lost more weight very quickly.

There was always a variety of foods for the residents. I used to think that the quantum on the plates was more for a man than for smaller and older ladies. Margaret, however, was losing all interest in eating. She was more interested in sleeping. Sometimes I would feed Margaret her lunch while she had her eyes closed. It seemed too difficult for her to open them. As long as I put the food in her mouth she would happily chew and swallow. At other times though I would not try to feed her, so sleepy was she. If she did eat she would eat very little. She did retain her 'sweet tooth'. Dessert was always welcome, and she drank well.

As I indicated earlier, each day in the court brought its little events. You never could tell for sure what would happen on any one day. My diary of 4 January captures what could happen:

> *"At lunch Betty pinched my bum. I jumped and one of the other ladies almost fell out of her chair with laughter."*

Good old Betty was old enough to be my mother. Unfortunately for me I am tall. She showed little interest in shorter men. I often thought it would be safer for me if I walked around on my knees.

The women in the court all had their moments. I grew to know and to respect them all. It was a living example of the fact that dementia pays no respect to status or prior intellectual and/or artistic acumen.

When Margaret was asleep it was easy for me to take my leave. On 7 January I record what I felt when she was awake as I left.

> *"I found it hard to leave her she was so wide awake, had hold of my hand and did not want to let it go. I feel at times I am as lonely as she is, perhaps more so, but I can help myself. She reacts well when Diane speaks to her. They wink at one another. She will wash her own face at times and, if prompted, will give herself a drink if you place the glass in her hand."*

January 14 was one of those days when Margaret would say something coherent.

> *"Marg was in good form. I took her for an outing in her wheel chair. She walked so well for Diane today too. Marg tries to talk with me. As I was going she said quite distinctly, 'Oh, do you have to go?'"*

And again on 29 January:

> *"She woke just before lunch. Was wide awake when I left. She actually said very clearly, 'Bye, bye.' It was lovely. Then she asks, 'Going home now?' I have been smiling ever since. Love her so much."*

I really took great pleasure in any sign of rational brain activity in my Margaret. In a similar way I looked for her smile of recognition. It is strange to now admit that I would feel hurt when she smiled at others and did not smile at me. On a good day I would be on a high as on 4 February:

> *"I found her awake after 30 minutes. While she sleeps I just sit beside her and hold her hand. I love doing that. When she woke I gave her a milk coffee. We then went out to be with the group. She loves that when awake. Looks around and smiles a lot. She held my arm for 30 minutes too. She ate her lunch. I gave her one of her ice creams too. I wrote some good comments on Di, Louise, Rhonda & Rachael. I just know when Di is on.. Marg's room is so clean as too is she. Love it."*

I began to notice that Margaret was curling up her hands and arms across her chest. The visiting physiotherapist taught me a few exercises for Margaret to help release those muscles. I would do them daily for her arms, hands, legs and feet. She always loved having her feet massaged.

Margaret's birthday came due on 7 February. She was 67. Deep in my heart I sensed that it would be the last with me. I truly feel that she knew that too.

> *"Marg was asleep when I arrived. She would wake on occasion to look at me and smile. She then did something she has not done for a long, long time. I can't remember when. She actually leaned towards me and kissed me twice on the lips gently. I felt so strange about that but I loved it. On her 67th birthday that was her gift to me – just for a change – she was always giving."*

She had other visitors for her birthday. Her daughters came as their work permitted. Margaret's mother and her youngest sister were regular visitors also. Margaret was never left out of our extended family's social world. Yet even though I was with her each day I would miss her presence at home. My reflection of 12 February was:

> *"I have been feeling very emotional in the past day or two. Perhaps it is from re-reading the letters I wrote to Marg in 1965 (all 158 of them). I gave so many assurances of my love, of its depth, of my guarantee to care for her, that I continue to recall the times when I was other than caring. It hurts to think that I may have offended her and that I cannot ask her forgiveness nor talk to her. She has been such a strong influence on my life I am really lost without that, hard though it may be for me to admit it. As I left her today, sitting askew to the left in her wheelchair, I cried. I hate seeing her as she is. As she was toileted I could see her hips were gone, her bottom was limp and sagging – all muscle tone had gone. In many ways she is now firmly in God's hands. We used to pray a lot to Mary. I trust she now keeps Marg enfolded in her arms. How I would want to do that but cannot. What is it to live without the one I lived for most of my life. God it is lonely here at times."*

Margaret weighed just 47.9 kilos. She was approximately 56 kilos when she entered Nandeebie in July 2005. I had to take the recently purchased size 14 trousers home and replace them with size 10. Thank God for Miller's! She was no longer taking Aricept as their usefulness had long run its course. She was eating irregularly, sleeping a lot more, and her spasms were more frequently. She would sometimes forget to chew when food was in her mouth. Little wonder that my emotions were raw.

> *"Have shed a number of tears again today. I just feel so lonely without my Marg. There are so many things I would want to say to her, but up front would be my wanting to ensure she knows she is always the love of my life. I try to thank God for the gift she has been for me. Even now she is a gift. I get to visit, to feed, to care for her in so many ways. In this way she is still the way for me to find my way into heaven. I assume, with confidence, she has one leg in there already."*

I felt this way for many days. My mood was not helped by watching a movie called "The Notebook" in which a young woman had Alzheimer's. There were too many parallels with events in our life. Still, life went on. The ongoing banter at lunch time had to bring a smile to your face. When I bought a cream cake for our elderly nurse and resident, Maisie, I could not help but feel good.

> *"Cost only $5. She was delighted and made me cut the first slice for her."*

Maisie's action was a far cry from that of good old Betty who was forever following me around the court. Retiring to Margaret's room was not necessarily a safe haven.

> *"Betty was a buggar today. I dislike her touching me. When one resident was coughing badly she called out, 'Get it up ducky, it could be a gold watch.'"*

At times my poor Margaret would be caught in the crossfire of the little spats that went on in the court amongst the residents. Much of the angst arose from some of the ladies wandering in and out of other residents' rooms. This was not appreciated by some and so the verbal stoushes would erupt. On one occasion one of the ladies got stuck into Margaret as she lay helpless in her regency chair. Margaret's eyes grew wide with wonderment and a little fear. Later the lady tried to apologise. She did seem to know what she had done to Margaret. I asked her not to enter Margaret's room in the future.

During the month of March there was no relief for Margaret from her spasms and her lean. Her carers would try to make her as comfortable as possible in her regency chair through the use of cushions. Sometimes her head would be tilted backwards at such an angle that there was a great strain on her neck muscles. In this position swallowing was very difficult. I would support her head and gently move it forwards to try to relax the muscles, especially at meal times.

Meal times were a growing concern. Margaret was so sleepy she would miss breakfast and/or lunch many times. It seemed like every second day I was with her she spent most of the time sleeping. When she was very tired and sleepy it was too dangerous to try to feed her. Even on a good day she would eat no more than half of that prepared for her. As I mentioned earlier there were supplements for her and I also kept strawberry and chocolate milk in the refrigerator for her. She liked them and the ice-cream and sweets I had for her too. Whenever there was an opportunity I would give her something from this private supply. I know the facility would have supplied these for me had I requested it, but it gave me pleasure to supply these few things for her.

Margaret's weight had fallen further at her monthly weigh in on 19 March. She was now 45.5 kilos which was some 10 kilos less than what she was when she entered Nandeebie. In the old terms this represented a loss of one and a half stone. So on 3 March I record:

> *"I was shocked to see my little 'Tweetie' sitting on her shower stool having a shower. She seemed to enjoy the shower and was not embarrassed by my presence. In fact I got a great smile from her. She looks so thin though and totally dependant. How far removed is this from my beautiful young bride of 40 years ago."*

I keep highlighting little things that occur that were so joy filled. Except for my diary I may have forgotten them as the painful experiences were the most powerful. On 5 March one of the carers was holding Margaret after her toileting subsequent to lunch. The carer, in her usual gruff but loving way, asked if I would like to give my wife a hug. While I think Margaret wondered what the hell was going on, I held her in my arms. That was a very emotional moment for me. Nicole had a way of knowing what I would like to do at times. Then on the next day:

> *"Marg was sleeping. She slept until about 11.30. I bent over her and asked her for a kiss. She actually gave me one. There is little warmth in her tiny lips though. I have been asking God to talk to her and tell her I love her, always have and always will. I have a deep, deep desire to tell her that once more, and know that she hears and understands."*

Margaret's doctor visited her regularly. He was pleased with the state of her general health. Her problems with swallowing were certainly related to her disease, but, to be on the safe side, Annette decided that it may be good for a speech therapist to observe Margaret at one lunch period. She did so on 15 March and confirmed the problem appeared rather to do with the brain's dysfunction than anything else. If this became more serious I would be faced with a decision about force feeding Margaret through tubes. Annette showed me the tubes available and talked me through the process involved. I was emotionally a wreck at the very thought of what it would entail. I wanted to consult with my family, but I knew in my heart that I would not force Margaret through that ordeal. I felt sure she would not want it either. Little wonder that my diary of 9 March records:

> *"I am a mess. I have just come home from having a lovely tea with Maree and family. I thought I would tell them of Margaret's problems with swallowing without great emotion, but, fool that I am, I could not. I cried – sobbed really – and Maree held me and cried too. I hate being a burden to them. They have enough to contend with but I just feel so alone and so deeply sad. I cried all the way home. I sit and hold my beautiful wife's hand at Nandeebie and I cry while she sleeps. Tears are just under the surface all day. I just can't seem to control them. I do miss having*

> *a support - Marg was always my support. That she could starve to death just makes me so sad. I find myself praying to Jesus to take her quickly. He obviously wants her back, why else this terrible disease. Why not then take her. She was asleep when I arrived today. She woke partially to have her hair cut. She was leaning very noticeably today too. She would not eat much for me. She did not have her breakfast either. She looks so frail. I get jealous of the beautiful smiles she gives to others. She seems not even to notice I am there. It hurts. I love her so deeply. Lord only knows what life will be like without her being with me."*

Whenever possible I continued to take Margaret out into the pergola or around the grounds. She loved these ventures, at least for a while, and then she would doze off again. If anyone tried to treat her as if she were normal, Margaret would do her best to interact with them in return. My son–in–law, Michael, always treated Margaret that way as I record on 31 March:

> *"Michael and Sean were there before me. I think it is beautiful the way Mike sits there and just talks to Marg – tells her about the kids and all. Every so often she will smile at him. They are moments to treasure."*

I would always try to interact in that way with Margaret as I note of one of her typical sleepy days on 1 April:

> *"She went to sleep soon after I arrived. I took her out to the pergola. Such a lovely day. We sat out there and I prattle on to her. She opens her eyes on occasion, gives me a smile, then off to sleep again. She did eat most of her lunch then went to sleep again."*

The following day I had one of those treasured yet highly emotionally charged experiences. I arrived as Margaret was to be showered. I volunteered to assist. She showed no embarrassment and enjoyed the play of the warm water over her emaciated body.

> *"I feel so deeply a sense of her loss. She is totally defenceless, totally reliant upon others to look after her. I brushed her hair and fed her some of her breakfast."*

When Margaret had her flu needle in April, I wondered where they found a place to inject her. She was having supplements twice a day at this point, yet was so thin and frail.

I had a full day at Nandeebie on 7 April after being accepted as a volunteer. I was helping with the filing and archiving that was necessary for the residents. On these days I would spend time with Margaret until she finished her lunch. She would normally have a sleep period after lunch. I then went to do my filing and returned later in the afternoon to assist Margaret with her evening meal at 5pm.

> *"She ate her soup, half a piece of bread, a little egg and some custard. When I told her I was going she reached out and held my hand. I feel so terrible when I have to leave her. Lord only knows how she feels. Please God watch over her always for me."*

Getting Margaret to open her mouth to take her tablets involved a struggle often and also some ingenuity. I was intrigued one day to see Cath put the crushed tablets in some ice cream. Margaret took them without any trouble. When I struggled desperately to have Margaret eat at least some of her lunch for me, I would have a cold washer close at hand to wipe her face hoping to keep her awake. I usually lost these battles to sleep. Margaret now weighed 44 kilos.

At Nandeebie I was of the belief that I hid my emotional self from the people I interacted with each day. I should have known that the wonderful women that care for people in nursing homes were far more aware than I thought. On 16 April:

> *"After lunch with Marg – she ate most – I was sitting holding her hand and that Nicki asked if I was OK, then handed me a box of tissues. Somehow she sensed or knew what I was feeling and the feeling will just not go away."*

On 18 April I was approached about moving Margaret out of the dementia specific court. There had been a couple of deaths so places were available in one of the high care courts. Such a move was not simple and I wanted to take the family's thoughts into consideration.

Margaret was very much at ease with the majority of her carers. I loved the persons and the personalities that made up the community of Kanaipa. The secure nature of the grounds around the court was ideal for the grandchildren who visited regularly. However, we had been part of the Nandeebie family long enough to know that there were others desperate to find a secure environment for their loved ones. For some months Margaret had not been mobile and was confined to her regency chair. It was not all that difficult to ultimately convey to Robyn and Annette that we would move to Kyogle, one of the high care courts.

It was not long after this that I had an intense spiritual moment with my loving wife. It was a Sunday, 23 April.

> *"Got out to see Marg just before 10am. Marg was awake. Pam told me she had eaten a good breakfast. I hosed the pergola then took her outside with me. I sat and talked to her for some time. She would close her eyes but listen. At times she would nod agreement. Once I closed my eyes and prayed to Jesus asking, that since He came to me in communion last night at mass, would he allow me to pass that on spiritually to my beautiful wife who loved mass and communion maybe even more than I. I felt Marg's hand tighten on my hand and I opened my eyes to see her staring intently at me. Make of it what you will, but for me it was a very special and spiritual moment."*

The following day was my final 'bun' Monday at Kanaipa. I would often buy a large cream filled bun or two on Mondays for the residents. They devoured it, helped usually by the carers. The only person who would not eat any was my Margaret.

Margaret's legs were beginning to curl up at the knee. My guess is that without regular stretching they may have eventually moved into a foetal position and remained there. With the guidance of the physiotherapist I had several stretching exercises that I would do daily with her.

The wall mounted air conditioner that I had installed for Margaret in her room at Kanaipa was moved to her new room. Nandeebie agreed to meet half the cost for me. The move ended up costing nothing other than my undertaking to pray for a month for the personal needs of John, the man who re-installed it for us. For him it was a labour of love, a Christian act seeking no human reward. He was not a member of my church but of the one attended by my sister Colleen. What an example such people are to us all.

Early in May Margaret had the first signs of a pressure sore. It became very difficult to manage the thinner she grew. It was the aim of all staff at all levels to ensure she had no pain and that the pressure sore be healed. A regime of moving her every two hours was put in place. A soft lamb's wool rug was also placed under her while she was in her regency chair. That rug was a legacy from dear Molly, a fellow resident, who had died some little time earlier.

I wished to continue to take Margaret into the fresh air as much as possible. Her leaning and her spasms made outings in her wheel chair almost dangerous. I asked about strapping her into the chair.

> *"I asked about a strap to hold Marg in but that is classified as a restraint so would need a doctor's OK."*

By 12 May the doctor had approved a restraint for the wheel chair only. In the end I never got to use it. The lifting from her regency chair to the wheel chair was just too distressing for her. I grew confident enough to be able to push her regency chair anywhere in the facility that I wanted to take her. Margaret was safe in it. A special event was put on for mothers on 11 May.

> *"They had a special lunch for Mothers Day. Marg was one of seven residents in a regency chair. I fed her. After lunch an elderly lady called me over. She asked if it was my mother – a common error – I told her it was my wife. She then paid me a great compliment by saying how beautiful it was to see me minister to her as I did. You just never know what effect you are having on others. Marg ate most of her lunch then slept."*

In recording our journey with Alzheimer's I continued to be aware of how the good moments in the journey are weighed down by the not so good. Carers, in my opinion, must try to recognise the good days and bask in them as I did on 13 May:

> "I took her out to the pergola at about 11am. I sat beside her with my arm around her and massaged her back. She seemed to enjoy that and I talked to her. Her eyes were really alive for a good time. She would nod to me at times too. I really loved that small window to her today. It does not happen all the time but, when it does, it is so precious."

Margaret was no longer able to straighten her legs to stand. The move to Kyogle had gone sweetly. Her carers voiced their concerns about walking her. On 24 May:

> "I asked Cath about her. Her bowels have not been functioning too well it seems. They also are concerned for Marg's safety when walking her. They trialled using the pixel (a lifting machine) and it worked in so far as Marg held on to it. They will use it only when a nurse is on call."

I was amazed how well my thin little Margaret could hold on as the pixel lifted her weight for her. It was not long though before the sling hoist (my description) had to be used, as she could no longer use her arms to lift or steady herself.

As had been the case when we first moved to Kanaipa, there was a settling in period to negotiate at Kyogle Court. Being in the court each day made me aware of little things I did not want to be left unaddressed. There had been a change of clinical nurse from Annette to Sharyn. She was quite open to meeting regularly to discuss issues and to seek solutions. I was never made to feel unwelcome or that I was being a nuisance. There were no recriminations if constructive criticism or genuine concerns were raised. I observed that changes were implemented. I say again that the family primary carer is the advocate for the resident and is honour bound to act as such.

What I knew Margaret would want for herself and what I would want her to have became the benchmark for me in determining what was acceptable and what was not. It was then unacceptable to find her mouth had not been sponged clean after a meal. I always did this after every meal when I fed her. It was unacceptable to have her remain in clothes she may have soiled by spilling some of her food. It was unacceptable that there were significant changes in her medications without my being at least informed. It was unacceptable that she not be showered daily as set out in her care plan. As her health and strength deteriorated that was reviewed. These were the types of issues I would take forward as Margaret's advocate.

There was a young music therapist who came to the court each week for an hour. I would wheel Margaret in to be part of Alison's session. Though Margaret loved music, more often than not the need for sleep won over. Her snoring would often punctuate any silences in the common room. When she was awake, Margaret would interact very positively with Alison as she sang to her. At Kyogle, if Margaret was awake, I:

> "Just sat with her. Manipulated her feet, arms and legs. Gave her a drink of iced coffee. Later she ate well for lunch."

At other times as on 9 June:

> "Marg was wide awake for me today. We held hands and 'talked'. I tell her all that is going on in the family. She seems to listen, though at times gets a far away look. She got sleepy at lunch time as usual."

I was rather pleasantly surprised when on 10 June one of the regular carers approached me with a compliment:

> "Belinda told me she loves the way I just talk to Margaret as if she were able to be part of the conversation. Says she rather finds herself talking at the residents."

There were times when Margaret would still show signs of a life within that she could seldom express. Marg stayed asleep all the time I was with her on 14 June but:

> "Cath told us earlier this morning Marg was laughing, really laughing. She seemed to be tickled by things Mary was saying to her."

Mary was quite a character and confined to a regency

chair also. Later in June Margaret remembered my name. I was not there when she did.

> *"Marg had just been changed when I arrived. Knocked her breakfast all over herself. Cath told me she said, 'No Vince, No Vince' while they were changing her."*

If Margaret's spasms grew to be sharp and obviously distressing to her, she would be given some Risperodone. It usually did reduce the severity of the spasms. My anxiety levels rose each time Margaret would refuse to eat much of her lunch. I tried to force the spoon through her teeth as she clenched them like a child who was refusing to eat what you had prepared for them. On 17 June:

> *"Later I tried it on myself at home. Realise now it could hurt her mouth. Will not do it in the future. Her only way of saying I don't want it is to not open her mouth. She drinks OK so I can always give her a meal that way."*

Towards the end of the month Margaret developed a very sore toe. It was inflamed. Her head was bending backwards making eating and swallowing very difficult. I had begun to give a series of personal development seminars to staff who showed some interest. Filing was always there to do and there were other little jobs to be done as they became obvious to me. I felt fully part of the Nandeebie family. Nothing however took away the ache I had for my girl though, as I mention on 28 June.

> *"Do little things where and when I can. Back to help Marg with her tea. Gee I love her. I think even now she is so beautiful and I miss her presence here with me. Life can indeed be cruel and I am sure that nobody knows what I am going through. I certainly don't know what Marg is going through."*

I was spoilt at Kanaipa by having access to a pergola for Margaret. At Kyogle there was a small concrete apron outside the central doorway. It was overcrowded when there were two or three regency chairs there. Nonetheless I would wheel Margaret out into the fresh air each day.

The roller coaster of periods of sleep and wakefulness continued throughout July. The glare from the bright sunlight I thought may have been giving Margaret a headache. I resurrected her old sunglasses and they worked a treat. They made it difficult to tell if she was awake though. The septic toe I mentioned earlier had eventually to be pierced to relieve the swelling. When Cath did that all the complaining that came from my girl was a little cry of pain. The healing process was slow but sure thank God.

Margaret developed a habit of raising her tongue toward the roof of her mouth when I was feeding her. It was a rather tricky manoeuvre to get the spoon over her tongue before she raised it. I did not read this as a sign that she did not want to eat. It was another expression of the disease. No matter how hard we all tried to have her eat well, her weight was now down to 40 kilos.

From one day to the next I was never sure in what direction her body would be bent. On 5 July:

> *"Marg was awake. She looked bent today, almost in a Z position while in her regency chair. She ate well. I cradled her in my arms for 15 minutes at one stage. She really nestled there and closed her eyes, quite at peace. Really broke me up. I can easily count her ribs from the back these days."*

I began the search for a suitable tilt-in-place wheelchair for Margaret. I wanted to be able to take her out around the grounds. It was far too difficult for me pushing a regency chair. Tilt-in-place wheelchairs were very expensive. It took so long to sort out price and details that I eventually dropped the idea. My need to take her for a ride around the grounds was one thing; the pain to her of being lifted from regency to wheelchair was another.

Margaret's updated care plan was signed off on 17 August with only a few slight amendments. It was not part of the care plan but Cath and I thought that for Margaret to have a little glass of sherry when her spasms were bad may help her to settle, and thus not have to take the Risperodone. On the first occasion I tried this she slept like a baby. She was no drinker, but did like a small sherry in the past. When next I gave her a small drink she remained wide awake, but it did calm her somewhat.

August saw the birth of our fifth grandchild. Megan had another little girl. She was named Margaret after her grandmother and would be called Maggie. I tried to explain all this to my Margaret. I got the impression she at least knew something grand had happened.

I had a chance to talk with Margaret's physiotherapist. Her legs, especially the left one, was so bent that I wondered how much stretching to do. His advice:

"Good to continue but don't overdo and hurt her."

Many years earlier Margaret had had a couple of operations on the toes of her left foot. They had been left straight by those operations, but now one of them had been somehow bent over. For a second time it became inflamed. By 29 August it needed to be opened to release the inflammation. It began to heal after that.

As August came to an end our journey with Alzheimer's was also coming to its end. A long diary note of 27 August says:

"When I got to Margaret this morning I noticed that she had a 'wet' cough. She looked a little distressed. I asked Nicki about it. She brought the RN down. Seems Marg had been blue around the mouth earlier. They decided to give her oxygen. That was a bit of a farce as they had trouble locating the oxygen, then trouble putting it to work. They were going to suck stuff out of Marg's mouth, but could not get it to work. I was really upset internally. I know that statistically most Alzheimer patients die of pneumonia or some form of aspiration. They believed she had a little noise in her lungs. Dr had been contacted. Suggested hospital if no improvement."

This was a Sunday. On 28 August:

I could not wait to get to Nandeebie to check on Margaret. I ran into Cath first. She was on her way to a 3 hour assessment. Then saw Pat. She told me Marg was much better today. Indeed she was. She did have a lot of spasms, arms and legs going. She was not coughing. She ate well at lunch for me too."

The problem of the location of the oxygen supply was sorted out. I also confirmed that if Margaret had to go to hospital at any time I wanted her at either the Mater Private or the Greenslopes Private. Not much use in paying for health cover all your working life and then not using it. I do thank God that we never had to face that eventuality.

Earlier in the month I was occasionally aware of a rather peculiar odour about Margaret. As far as I could tell it was not a body odour. I noted also that she would grow very agitated when left in certain positions in her regency chair. Investigation showed that there was redness on a section of her rear that was the beginning of a 'bed sore'. The regime of having her moved every couple of hours was recommenced. On 30 August:

> "Had a good discussion today with Sharyn and Cath re Margaret. We covered the need for her to be moved regularly in her regency chair. I have not seen that done while I am with her. Also the pressure tear she has. We discussed the smell about her at times. With my OK they will get the Dr to do a test for cervical cancer although there is no vaginal flow of any kind at the moment. Told of my planned week away. Told me to go and enjoy. Marg is in the last stages of the disease, but not in its last stages. I was thankful for their time and attention. They appear to be appreciative of my bringing matters to their notice."

Then the next day:

> "When I got to Nandeebie there was a little shock for me. Marg was in bed sleeping soundly. Jan found her bottom to be a little worse than yesterday so they decided a day in bed would do Margaret the world of good. Far easier to keep her off her sore spot. She had eaten her breakfast. Sharyn told me when she saw Marg early in the morning, Marg was awake and talking. When she asked Marg what she would like she said quite clearly, 'Get up please'. At another occasion when getting her set up for breakfast Sharyn asked Marg was there anything else, to which Marg replied, 'A little higher please'. Sharyn was gob smacked. Marg slept most of the morning, had lunch in bed too."

Margaret's general health grew worse during the month of September. I believe there would have been times when she aspirated, that is took food or drink into her lungs. It was almost inevitable that that would happen at some stage. She was finding it difficult to determine what she should do with a mouth full of liquids. Sometimes she would try to chew the liquids and at other times she would swallow a little at a time. It was hard to tell whether or not she had swallowed the lot.

The pressure tear was not healing. Its location made it extremely difficult to attach the patches that would normally help in the healing process. Medicinal honey was tried and it too did little to alleviate the growing problem. It was a time of some discomfort for my dear wife. Her only way to tell us of her discomfort was through her physical agitation. Once she was moved off the pressure point she would then relax and fall asleep.

From 3 September Margaret was back in her regency chair for part of the day. Her carers were meticulous about moving her every two hours. After lunch she would be hoisted onto her bed for her sleep.

Megan came down to see her mother with the littlest family addition, Maggie, on 4 September:

> *"Marg always gives Megan a great smile. We placed little Maggie in her arms and Marg held on with a look of delight in her eyes and face."*

I will always remain convinced that, even in the deepest part of her disease, Margaret was aware of the significance of some events. I wrote on 5 September:

> *"I took her outside and we sat and talked. There are times I feel she knows I am doing just that – talking to her. She responds by her looks and tries to say things and ask questions. She loves to hold my hand and she will gently stroke my arm. I get such a great buzz out of that. Have no idea what she is saying to me but we are in a weird sense 'communicating'."*

On another day when Megan was with me and she had Eliza and baby Maggie with her:

> "Cath took Maggie around to the residents. They all loved the experience. Marg was awake and came alive when she saw Megan. She was rather anxious for a time though and Cath wondered whether she wanted to hold the baby. Megan put Maggie on Marg's chest and Marg held her such that she would not let go. Marg's eyes told you how much this meant to her. I am sure she gets so frustrated that she cannot nurse & stroke the little one. She did settle markedly after the nurse."

A few weeks later I was discussing Margaret's well being with Cath when Margaret grew very angry. Her anger was so obvious that it shocked all of us present. I read that, as did we all, that she was saying to us, "Don't talk about me. Include me".

The disease had taken its final hold on my love. I began to sense deep within myself that there was not long to go in our journey. On 14 September I record:

> "I am never sure whether one should write when one's emotions are churned up. I had an overwhelming sense as I stood beside Marg's bed this afternoon and watched her poor little emaciated body lying there asleep that her time was not very long. I have been in tears ever since. She seems to be just fading away. I keep wondering how you can lose weight when you have none."

24 hours was a long time in our journey. I was never sure what to expect as I walked towards Kyogle. Margaret could look at death's door one day:

> "Marg looked unwell to me today. Her skin is yellowish. She has a wet cough too."

And then the next:

> "She seemed to enjoy everyone's presence. She had eaten a good breakfast I was told. I hated leaving her as she was still wide awake. I kissed her goodbye and said, 'I will see you tomorrow'. In her quiet little voice she said, 'Okay'. Boy it's hard."

I knew that it was not the right time for me to be away

from her as I had planned. She was weighed at 37.5 kilos on 23 September. If it was possible, she was eating less for me at lunch and looking for more and more sleep. The disease does that, but I felt that sleep also gave her some alleviation from the discomfort of her pressure tears and her lungs. When she would lie down she would develop a dry cough, so a nebuliser was used at night to help her rest.

The thinner Margaret became the more her large dark eyes seemed to stand out. Her beautiful eyes were always part of her attraction to me at least. Now I hated the way they would stare at me when I was leaving. They would have an appeal in them for me to stay with her. They haunted me then and they haunt me now. On 2 October:

"I left at 12.45 and her big black eyes watched me go."

Margaret's pressure tears were looking very red and raw by 5 October:

"After lunch I helped to put ointment on her sore bottom. I actually carried her from her regency chair to her bed. Her bottom looks so sore. Please God it gets better soon. It must be so uncomfortable for her yet she never complains my love. What an exemplar she remains for me."

To this day I can feel her little shell of a body in my arms. The hoist at that time was in use elsewhere and we did not know how long we would have to wait for it to be free. I picked her up in my arms. I remember that Margaret was as light as a feather. I really did not want to put her down once I had her in my arms. I was not to know it, but this would be the last time on this earth that I would hold her so.

On the following day I was asked if I would relax the need for Margaret to be showered each day. It was taking so much out of her that she was totally exhausted after the experience. She would be bed washed each alternate day. I agreed that this would be best for Margaret.

On 7 October Margaret was surprisingly alert. Maree with her daughter, Emer, was visiting then also.

> *"Marg was really alert by this time and gave Maree some beautiful smiles. I was so pleased as Maree seems to miss out. It was as if Marg knew her to be one of her children."*

My experience the next day is best captured in my diary note:

> *"At mass last night I had what I would call a religious moment. I was praying before mass and, as usual, my thoughts turned to our family, in particular my Margaret. I have been suggesting to God that while I accept the upshot of her disease is death, I don't believe she should have to suffer pain in her time left. I thought of Marg's life and I believe she was closer to God than I have ever been. While I am still a sinner, her Alzheimer's would mean for years she could not have sinned. I look forward to her being with God so that, selfishly, she may aid me in my journey there to be with her. I was so aware that all of us are God's children, that Marg has been God's gift to me these 41 years, and that that time approaches when He will want her to return to her home with Him. I had a very great sense, an insight maybe, that in her innocence in her disease, Margaret was already more with God than with me. I was not saddened by this thought and feeling. Rather did I feel joy and, to an extent, relief to know to whom she was going.*
> *Today I felt good about going to Nandeebie. I had cut a long stemmed rose, a Margaret rose, from our front garden to take to her. When I arrived there was a sombre tone. Marg was still in bed and she looked so frail and in pain. Cath told me Marg was doing it tough. Her pressure sores, now two, were not improving, rather they were worsening. She would/could not eat. A doctor had sent an authority to get pain relievers as a suppository. Her own doctor would be in tomorrow. She was flushed. She was moaning. Her body looks like a skeleton with a thin layer of skin over it. Of course I broke down. I will never be ready for the inevitable and my experience at mass made it all the more difficult. I rang Maree and cried yet again. Anne arrived later with Bernie and Helen. I just wanted to be alone with Marg but that would be very mean. Maree came up also God love them. Megan was at a christening. I did get Marg to drink a pro-form Milo for lunch. She was good for 30 minutes.*

> *When I left at 1.15 she was asleep but struggling with pain. I hope the next suppository works at 2pm. I have been breaking down all afternoon. I pray that God does not let her linger no matter what the pain of her going will mean for me. I feel like part of my inner self is being extracted. I would hope that that was so because in us, two really did become as one."*

That was Sunday. On Monday I was pale and sick to the core. My good friend, Joe, rang in the morning. He told me he had a premonition that he should ring. I headed off to Nandeebie early.

> *"Got there at 9.30. Marg was awake and wide eyed. Cath told me she did not sleep all night. I got the feeling Marg was scared to go to sleep. She gave me some great smiles today, thank God. Megan left at 11.15 or so. Marg began to have her breathing very shallow with heart racing. Dr came at 12.30. Said her lungs were filling. Asked if I wanted her in hospital. I said no. He believed that was best for her also. Nandeebie is her home. They have pain killers for her. She is in pain my poor love. Cath said even the carers have to deal with Marg as she now is. I really do think she is not long for this world. God wants her."*

I had to return home for an hour or so, but then returned to Nandeebie to sit with Margaret. She would not eat but did have half a glass of liquid:

> *"Left at 6pm. She closed her eyes finally when I kissed her goodnight."*

I would never see those beautiful eyes wide open again. The next day, 10 October 2006, would be Margaret's last day with us. Her family was so much part of her life that it was appropriate that God, in His wisdom and love, allowed us to be with her. Had she been able to open her eyes and focus, she would have seen us – her children (Maree, Megan and Anne), her grandchildren (Tom, Sean and Maggie), her son-in-law Michael, Anne's husband to be Richard, her mother Bernie and youngest sister Helen. She would have delighted in the life ongoing around her. As she breathed her last Megan sat feeding Maggie while Maree changed Sean's dirty nappy. Tears flowed throughout the morning. None was as moving as those that ran down Margaret's own pale cheeks as we sat close by talking to her for the last time.

My final diary note during the life of my greatest friend, lover, wife and mother to our children was penned late on 10 October 2006. My memory was affected by grief.

"I was awake when the phone rang at 5.20am today 10/10/06. Angela suggested that it was time for me to come in. I rang the girls, had a quick breakfast and was there by 6.30. They told me she had had a bad night – 7 times needed a change, almost choked herself, shaking in pain, etc. Now she was peaceful though her breathing was so laboured. Her eyes were only half opened and unmoving. She was seeing nothing. Her hands and feet were cold, but her head hot. Catherine gave her an oxygen feed to help. The family arrived and we spent the day watching and waiting. Staff were excellent with many in tears. Fr Peter came at 9am and gave Marg a final blessing and anointing. At mid morning Cath and Bronwyn washed and changed Marg. Her breathing was shallow and they were terrified she may die while I was out of the room. She struggled on yet again only with few breaths. I tried to tell her it was Ok to go to God. After lunch all left the room except for myself. Marg seemed to relax. Dawn was with me when I was aware she stopped breathing and that guttural 'death rattle' was heard. She finally had gone to God. No doubt Mary greeted her and led her to her Father in heaven. We stayed on until the funeral directors came to collect her. She was wrapped in a sheet and then plastic, strapped in and finally her face covered. I helped in the process. It will be with me always."

The journey we had taken together from 1997 had reached its climax, but the journey unfortunately had not ended. There was Margaret's final public farewell to celebrate her life, after which has followed such deep grief that words fail me. Even as I recall all the events so far recorded here, my body is racked with such a deep sense of loss. I actually do feel as if part of me has truly died. My continuing personal journey through the process of grieving is just that - a personal journey - still far from over.

Chapter 10

Epilogue

Farewell Margaret

*I*n one sense the role of the carer has come to an end with the death of the sufferer. The person being cared for is no longer present physically. In another sense the carer has yet to complete a number of tasks - the public farewell and all the legal niceties For Margaret we were able to organise her funeral to take place in a few days. Family support was again exceptional.

The night following Margaret's death I could not sleep at all. The next day was very draining emotionally and physically. I wrote on 11 October:

> "Only 1 hour's sleep. Up at 3am to write my eulogy. Girls were so great today my darling Margaret you would be so proud of them. Many phone calls and much work done on the funeral arrangements. Hope you my love enjoy our attempt to celebrate your life and journey, not that it all matters much to you as you are in your Father's House. Your job now my Margaret Mary Bernadette is to ensure we all get there to be eternally with you. Goodnight my sweetheart. As Megan says, 'Love you lots'."

Margaret's funeral was held at St James, Coorparoo on 13 October 2006. We had been married there 41 years earlier. I was totally astounded at the size of the congregation. The church was filled to overflowing. It spoke volumes for the high regard in which she was held by so many whose acquaintances she had made. The Archbishop of Brisbane attended and performed the final farewell. My girls wrote a letter to their mother which Megan read at the ceremony. What a treasure they are. This is what they had to say.

Dear Mum,

We got the phone call today. The call we knew was inevitable but prayed would never be made. You slipped away from us so quickly in the end. It's hard to accept we'll never lay eyes on your beautiful face again in this life, never see that glorious smile, and never meet your intense gaze. We'll never forget you.

As a kid it was always pretty easy to pick you out in one of our drawings. Dad was a bit tricky! Normally you had to look for the stick figure with brown pants pulled up too high and a face sporting long sideburns or a Merv Hughes moustache (it was the 70s!). But with you all we had to do was add some curly black hair and glasses to a smiley face!

Our promise to you, Mum, is that we'll make sure our children – your grandchildren – are able to draw you just as easily in body and in spirit the way we remember you – the way you should be remembered.

Our memories of you are so clear, yet sadly so selective. We wish we could remember more, that we'd taken more care to savour every moment we had as mother and daughter.

You were our friend and confidante; our disciplinarian and mentor; but importantly you were our wise teacher and guide. How we love you for that.

We'll tell our children about how funny grandma could be. We'll tell them of your intelligence; your deep love of learning and language, and how much you cherished the opportunity you had to become a uni student later in life. I remember so vividly sitting next to you in Mayne Hall at the University of Queensland on the day we both received our Bachelor of Arts degrees in 1991. How proud we were of you for having the courage to go back to complete high school with such distinction, and then to complete a Bachelor of Arts degree with such aplomb. We still envy your ability to summarise a 1500 word essay in just one sentence!

We'll tell them of your ability to surprise and to delight us; to burst into song at the drop of a hat. We'll teach our children to emulate grandma in the way they present themselves to the world. You were such a lady. You taught us by your constant example to treat every person with dignity and respect, to be polite, humble and gracious even to an enemy; and that there is a time and a place for every thing.

Mum, the life you lived is the example we try to follow in our lives with our partners and children. Although as typical teenagers we were often embarrassed at the sight of our parents holding hands in public, what greater love story could there be than your lifelong journey with dad. Your devotion to him is unsurpassed, and boy, has he shown the depths of his love for you, especially in recent years. You'd be so proud of him, Mum. There is no doubt that your marriage has guided us in choosing our partners.

Above all else though, Mum, it was your devotion to us, your daughters – Maree, Megan and Anne – that is your greatest legacy. Often the lives of mothers who stay home to look after their children are discounted by outsiders and even by their own children – but not yours. We realise (particularly now, having children of our own) how much of your life was aimed at giving us the best of everything and every possible experience and opportunity - and for that we are eternally grateful. You were *always*, always there for us - whether it was in simple ways like:

- Coming home from school to find freshly squeezed orange juice and Sao's with tomato and cheese laid out for afternoon tea.
- Taking us to athletics training, to tennis lessons and to competitions, sometimes all in one day

Or at the major events in our lives:

- Waking up to find you at our bedside after surgery
- Preparing for Maree and Michael's wedding
- Guiding us in our studies and delighting in our triumphs, whether on the sporting field or in our professional lives.

It is this deep devotion and love that we treasure and are now trying to replicate in our own families.

Oh, Mum, we knew that Alzheimer's would rob us of

you one day. But one of the terrible things about this disease is that with each stage of deterioration, with each loss of a skill (no matter how minor) over the last 7-8 years our hearts would break and re-break because we knew we were losing you piece by piece.

Many people didn't understand your suffering and you were abandoned by some when you most needed them. But til the end we know that even through the haze of the disease you knew and loved us and our children.

What really hurts is that we've missed out on so much together in our adult lives:
- Alzheimer's had taken hold of you by the time our children were being born
- When I got married
- When Anne met Richard

To not have access to your experience, guidance and knowledge during these last years has been tremendously painful for us girls. But we know from your expressions, from the tears that ran from your eyes (even on your last day) or the simple touch of your hand when you could still move them, that on some level you were always there for us and in our corner. And we know that our love for you also got through.

There has been a particular song by Elvis Costello that I've played to myself over the years that reminds me so much of you. It's simply titled "She" and it could well have been written for you.

For my part, each time I tried to read my eulogy I would break down. On the night before the funeral I recalled that one of Margaret's roles was to be my critic. Every speech I made during my working life she would listen to and critique for me. I took the photograph we had selected to go on her coffin and I read it to her. I did not break down once. So on the day of the funeral I did just that. I took her photograph with me and talked to her smiling face. I had little trouble delivering the eulogy that morning.

During our journey together with Alzheimer's I had experienced moments of deep grief. The disease strips the one so loved of most of the abilities we all take for granted in our daily living. As the prime carer I watched this day by day and I grieved for myself as well as for my beloved. In that grieving process Margaret was nevertheless still physically with me. I could reach out and touch her, stroke her hair, massage her legs and back, feed her, hold her, talk with her, etc. The grief now was different. It hurt from the depth of my soul. Like so many others, I have still to pass through the process of her finally departing.

I can best bring to a close the recording of our marvellous journey of love for one another, as we faced the inevitable outcome of Alzheimer's, by repeating what I wrote in the depths of my grief as Margaret's eulogy.

Each person's journey through life is truly unique. For 41 years of her 67 years on this earth it was my privilege and honour to be an integral part of Margaret Mary's journey. Our journeys were so entwined that it was and is hard for me at times to separate them. Really I don't want to separate them. Their conjoined nature, two vines that look like one to the casual observer, is my image of our covenant to become one body and one spirit in Christ through our marriage.

I would like this morning simply to share with you some insights into the person who was truly 'my better half'.

Margaret was born in Innisfail on the 7th February 1939 to Bernie and Eddie Clarke. She was the first of their seven children all of whom are here today. Bernie, who is with us here, was my mother's great friend through their school years in Rockhampton where they attended the Range Convent. In fact my mum, Ronnie, was Bernie's bridesmaid. Margaret grew into a beautiful young woman who loved ballroom dancing, Joan Sutherland, and singing in the Brisbane Girl's Choir. I first met her when as kids we were both living in Mackay. Later she would stay at our home in Sackville Street Greenslopes for a short time when she came to Brisbane to work before the family could follow. From afar, as a teenager, I thought she was truly beautiful, she thought I was a gangly pest.

I had entered the Augustinian Order after finishing high school in 1958. By late 1963 I knew I had to leave specifically because I just could not get thoughts of Margaret out of my head.

I had no idea whether she was still alive or whether she was single or married. When I saw her I knew immediately that I loved her. Margaret would later reveal to me, that on the day that I had decided to leave the Order, she was finishing a retreat and had an overwhelming feeling that something good was to happen to her. I always took that to mean that I was the something good. The hand of God has always been with us in our journeying through life together.

We were married here at St James on 11th December 1965. It was a warm though muggy day and when we reached the reception hall the beer had run out. Some of the little money we had allocated to a honeymoon had to be used to save the day. We travelled to Bailey's Motel at Noosa for our honeymoon, arriving late in the afternoon. My theological wisdom and laziness was able to argue well that we did not have to travel to find a mass for the next morning. Let me tell you we were at mass on Sunday and no matter how many times I tried this argument when we travelled even overseas I don't think I ever once won.

Fr Heffernan was the parish priest in Nambour where we attended mass. He of all people was preaching on 'the good wife'. About the only thing that Margaret remembered was his saying that it would be a virtue of the good wife to be 'frugal but not mean'. That became a principle of operation for Margaret throughout our lives, and our girls still laugh at the way she tried to pass that on to them with varying degrees of success. I am sure it was behind the many trips to op shops she and her sister Mary made in the early years of our marriage.

We settled in Ipswich where I was teaching in 1966. Here we had the first of our three wonderful daughters, Maree Therese. We moved to 33 Devon Street Annerley in late 1968 as I was then teaching at Villanova. Our two other daughters Megan and Anne were born at the Mater. Margaret was so delighted to have daughters. It meant that she could sew for them and pass on all her many skills. They were the focus of her life. There was nothing she would not do for them. Yet above all I knew she was my best friend, my rock, my better half.

No matter what I was to do in life she was there with me. When I became director of catholic education I asked Margaret to help me exemplify a married lay leader in our church. That was to be a difficult task for one who wanted always to be anywhere but in the spotlight. She was my constant companion though, even through the most mundane of public functions. When the going got tough, as it did on a number of occasions, I recall Archbishop Rush ringing home and when I would answer he would say, "I can always talk to you Vince, I have rung to speak to Margaret," and so I would put her on the line. She would be walking ten foot tall for days afterwards. She had a great love and respect for Bishop James Cuskelly. On those few occasions when my language would get a little more colourful than usual about things in James's hearing, he would come over to me and say, "How on earth did you ever get such a lady like Margaret to marry you?" I too have wondered at the hand of God even in that. Bishop James was present for the opening and blessing of Carmel College at Thornlands. At the cutting of the commemorative cake I stepped forward and James told me and the crowd that he did not want me, but the woman who was always with me, Margaret, and so they cut the cake together. Marg was beaming with pride and a little embarrassment.

Margaret loved reading. She had a marvellous facility with words and she became our walking dictionary. I was always so impressed by her spelling ability. She never once showed envy at my needing to study for many years. However, when the time was right she went back to school and completed her senior at Coorparoo State High. She then became a uni student. She was in her element. She loved every minute of it. Her study regime was a thing to behold and at no stage did she leave off the many other calls on her time. I was in awe of her capacity to learn and to write. She graduated in Arts in 1991 with Megan and then went on to do a course in Library management. All the while she continued as a special minister at our church, she took communion to the sick and elderly and did her stint for meals on wheels, and even found time to be in the Christian Marriage Society where we, together, made a tape on communication in marriage to help young people.

By late 1997 there were growing signs that all was not right with Margaret. It was in her major strength, the use of language, that the signs appeared. By early 1999 our neurologist,

Dr John Cameron, confirmed that Margaret had the early onset of Alzheimer's disease. He told us it was rampant and would grow rapidly. I was devastated. I can only imagine the fear in Margaret at this news. She was aware what it meant and together we researched the possible outcomes.

But even through her suffering she would continue to teach me, to change me. Even Bishop James would, I think, be astonished at my new found patience and tolerance. They were virtues hard to come by for me. I am sure Margaret would not mind me sharing one little anecdote. As the disease progressed, I was called upon to do everything for us. As I would be sweeping the kitchen floor my Margaret would stand in front of the broom. She just wanted to be nearby. I would have to hold her hand and move her, but she would eventually get in the way again. Over time I grew to just laugh about it with her. It really did not matter.

This was a time in our lives of great change. I cared for Margaret at home until July 2005. She then needed assistance even in standing. It was only in the last few months of her time at home with me that it became too difficult to take Margaret with me to Saturday evening mass at St James. I recall with joy her response on receipt of communion which was to simply say "Thankyou" - what need "Amen". I also recall with love the worried look on Fr Johnny McGlone's face when I approached him with Margaret in tow at a Second Rite of Reconciliation. It certainly was strange to confess in front of your wife. Perhaps we broke the Diocesan Law by receiving absolution together.

There were times when I think we both felt like modern day lepers, but without the bell. Alzheimer's seems to frighten people. Yet, through her disease, we found true friendship – a small group outside our family who were at peace with Margaret in public and whose friendship I will always treasure. They know well who they are. It is amazing to me how powerful a force for good has been Margaret's disease over this period on our lives and the lives of many others. For my part, for example, it has drawn me closer to my sisters and brother than ever before. Also, while I have railed against God often, I have experienced His gentleness and care.

With the help of Megan, I had visited up to 14 Aged Care facilities seeking a suitable place for Margaret. I decided to call in 'The Big Guns' and so, for the first time in many years I prayed the 30 days prayer to our Blessed Mother Mary. We had visited Nandeebie and had been told that the normal waiting time could be up to 6 months. As in all Aged Care facilities it is unfortunate that a room becomes available usually on the death of one of the residents. Both Megan and I had felt that Nandeebie best suited Margaret's needs, but realised that her needs had to be met earlier than in 6 months. That night I finished the 30 days prayer and in the morning received a phone call from Nandeebie saying that a room had unexpectedly become available. Naturally we accepted because their aim was to make us part of their family while respecting our family. And in this they succeeded admirably. Here again we experienced the hand of God in our lives.

We celebrated our 40th wedding anniversary at Nandeebie in December last year. From then on Margaret's life was confined to a regency chair and her bed. Though her language skills had been taken from her earlier, she had another signature gift at this time – her beautiful smile. It truly would make your day. I can't really say enough about the care that Margaret, and indeed all of us, received from so many – from the nursing staff (Pat, Pam, Angela, Nicky, Christine, Annette, Robin, Sharon, Karen, Katrina) and particularly Catherine Sherlock. And from the carers who treated her with such respect and dignity (Dianne, Louise, Rhonda, Lorraine, Bronwyn, Mary-ann, Jan, Karen, Michelle and Debbie) and of course from her doctor of more than 30 years, Bill Lee and more recently Dr Colquhoun.

When you try to put down some thoughts about a loved one at a time like this, it certainly would be easy to exaggerate, so may I repeat a few thoughts penned this Tuesday by a family friend Rosetta Pignatelli, from Scotland. They say what I would want to say of Margaret. I quote, "Margaret was truly unique. I always thought that she was saintly. She was so quietly spoken, gentle, kind and thoughtful. A real lady. I have never met another person like her. She made me feel, and no doubt everyone that she met feel special to her. I remember so many times when we were chatting she seemed so genuinely interested in what I was saying. Not many people have these qualities, and if more people had, the world would be a lot nicer".

Finally, while I was at a conference for Principals in 1994 I wrote a note to Margaret, part of which I think captures my thinking today. It reads:

Postscript

Some 16 years have passed since the original print of this book. I have learned much over that period. In particular, the continuation of my life's journey has brought me to more fully grasp how important is the unfolding of life after the caring role has ceased i.e., post care.

Grieving took its course as it does for each of us who care for a loved one as they journey to their death. That process will vary with each carer. In my own case, I came to understand that genuine grief had been my companion while caring, for the seven years from Margaret's diagnosis to her death. In many respects her death was an answer to my prayer that she may be finally at peace in one of the many mansions Jesus said were made ready for his just followers. Margaret was finally home.

When Margaret died and the funeral personnel had readied her body to be taken from the nursing home to the hearse, I knew I had to go with them. This was my final journey with her, so to speak. I assisted with the covering of her face, an act that for me signified the closure of one part of my life's journey. I continued volunteering regularly at the nursing home, Nandeebie, for a couple of months after her funeral. That was ended when I baked 87 Christmas fruit cakes as gifts for each of the caring staff. I never returned.

That aside, the writing of this book was the other major step for me in gathering my thoughts and moving on. The writing was a process for me, to discover and articulate meaning arising from the seven years of my caring role. It would become a corner stone in my post care period.

Writing this book was a major catalyst for a new direction in my life. I had, at that time, no firm answer to the 'What Now?' ever present in my mind. I had my health, I wanted to be useful, and life was there to be lived. In the first instance the writing of the book was to inform my children and grandchildren of the journey Margaret and I had taken together. It was my daughters who saw that our story may be of help to many others called to care for someone diagnosed with dementia, particularly male carers.

By publishing the book, my aim was to perhaps encourage a few hundred people to access the book. Through the good work of my daughter, Megan, I was interviewed on our National Radio, the ABC Brisbane, by Madonna King who organized an interview with Richard Fidler on the very popular 'Conversation Hour'. The book sold well after that.

Book sales certainly were important to offset the cost of publishing. More importantly for my journey, the radio interviews were instrumental in my being invited as a guest speaker at a conference organized by the Alzheimer's Association of Queensland in the city of Toowoomba. I was pleased that I was able to face an audience and present well while controlling the emotions that were close to the surface as I outlined my caring journey. Other speaking invitations were to follow from organizations including OzCare and Alzheimer's Australia. Several were requests to share my caring role at other venues under the aegis of the Alzheimer's Association of Queensland's Dementia Support Officer, Lorrae Martin.

Months later, though neither of us were initially seeking a relationship, one developed and Lorrae and I married at the commencement of 2010. Love found me again. Lorrae's elderly mother had dementia. We cared for her needs until her death in a nursing home nearly 97 years.

A special interest we shared was the need for carers to have genuine respite from their caring role. To develop that interest together, we used our shared resources of knowledge, skills, lived experience, and finances. So, our first home together, "Carers Outlook", blessed in the name of the Sacred Heart, became a sanctuary within which carer respite could be offered, a place where we cared for carers for a short period. This we did for 10 years as volunteers, during which I estimate we had over 450 respite stays with us. When the Covid pandemic hit the world stage in 2020 we ceased to offer respite. What a privilege it was to serve so wide a variety of carers. Through them our own understanding of the caring role greatly expanded.

During our respite service in our home, we attended a networking meeting of dementia staff overseen by Ozcare. As Ozcare couldn't continue this facilation, we were asked to continue the facilitation of the Dementia Network Sunshine Coast in Queensland. We took that up as volunteers, and we continue that to this day. We extended the service to provide events for people diagnosed with dementia, their family carers and staff including five social mornings, an exercise group, dementia choir, aqua aerobics group, family carer support group and presentations. September is Dementia month so we have organized events like an ecumenical service, seminars and 5 Dementia Conferences with Mooloolaba TAFE gifting the use of its venue. TAFE, Caloundra RSL and many organizations and individuals entrust us with donations to organize the events. We have literally supported thousands along our journey. The organizational tasks are undertaken by Lorrae whose energy and enthusiasm for the support of carers and those they care for is amazing.

What I have learned in the last 16 years is that we, the post carer group, need to plan ahead and be open to the opportunities that come our way post care. It is part of the process of finding meaning in life following a major disruption along the way. We need to be aware that opportunities arise at any time. These opportunities are gifts to be grateful for.

None of what we have accomplished would have been possible without an attitude captured in 'Carpe Diem' – Seize the Day. When opportunities, no matter how small they seem at the time, present themselves, post carers should strive to be open to how they may give new meaning to one's life.

Let the past inform the future, but don't let it dominate. In my experience, carers do tend to put their own lives on hold while they care for the other. However, each person's life is itself important and calls to be lived well.

If I have advice to give to those who are traversing the carers' role, it is to take time to care for yourself. Noone will provide the same dedicated and love-filled care that you do. It is imperative to not die on the job and so you must prioritize your health care and take respite. Likewise, as most carers will outlive the one being cared for, be wise enough to give time and energy to those parts of your life which will enable you to cope with life after the caring, particularly relationships with family and close friends. We are a relational animal, one whose emotional stability rests greatly on initiating and nurturing treasured relationships.

Dementia taught me that life is precious.

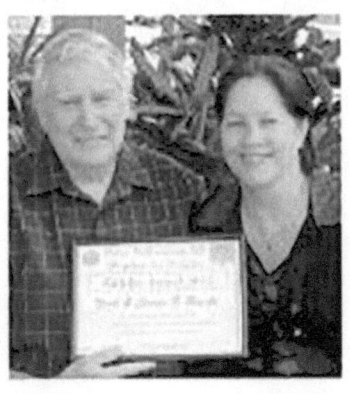
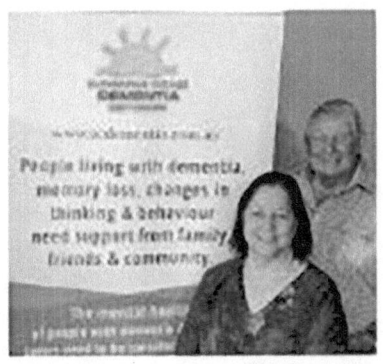

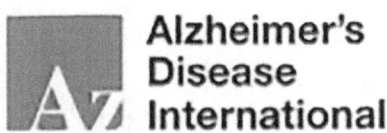
https://www.alzint.org/
Email: info@alzint.org
Tel: +44 20 79810880

Glossary

ACAT   (Aged Care Assessment Teams)

    Information under My Aged Care – www.myagedcare.gov.au or 1800 200 422

Aged Care Information Line

    www.seniors.gov.au   1 800 500 853

Alzheimer's Australia rebranded as Dementia Australia

    – 24 hr. Helpline 1800 100 500

Arrythmia

    Irregular heart beat

Cat Scan

    Computer Tomography Imaging - an X-ray. Can detect and determine the size and location of anatomical abnormalities such as tumours, lesions, blood clots and bone defects.

Centrelink

    An Australian Government Statutory Agency www.servicesaustralia.gov.au/centrelink

Commonwealth Carers Resource Centre

    There is one in each State and territory Capital City. 1 800 242 636

Currently Available Medications (non-exhaustive list)
Acetylcholine Esterase Inhibitors

Aricept (Donepezil)
Exelon (Rivastigmine)
Reminyl (Galantamine)
(Available on Pharmaceutical Benefits Scheme. Usually for mild to moderate sufferers. Dependent on improvement of cognitive skills measured by the Mini Mental State Examination.)
NMDA Receptor Antagonists.
Ebixa (Memantine) - relatively new for moderate to severe

EEG (Electroencephalogram)

> It measures the electrical activity of the brain via electrodes applied to the scalp.

MASS

> Medical Aids Subsidy Scheme
> www.health.qld.gov.au/mass/information.asp

MRI

> Magnetic Resonance Imaging. Shows greater detail than X-ray, CAT scan, etc.

National Continence Helpline

> 1 800 330 066

Rheumatoid Arthritis

> Affects joints, especially hands, feet and knees. About 75% of sufferers are female. Joints become inflamed and painful.

Relevant Contacts

Organization	Contact Information	Website	Services Provided
Alzheimer's Foundation of America (AFA)	866-232-8484 / Text: 646-586-5283	alzfdn.org	Memory screenings, caregiver support, dementia care training.
National Institute on Aging (NIA)		nia.nih.gov	Research, publications, tips for caregivers and healthcare providers.
Administration for Community Living	1-800-677-1116	eldercare.acl.gov	Local resources for elder care, support for long-term care planning.
Dementia Society of America (DSA)	1-800-336-3684	dementiasociety.org	Education, local resources, and caregiver support programs for all types of dementia.
Cure Alzheimer's Fund (CAF)	781-237-3800	curealz.org	Funds research on understanding and preventing Alzheimer's disease.
Alzheimer's Research and Prevention Foundation (ARPF)	1-888-908-5766	alzheimersprevention.org	Education on brain health, prevention strategies, and holistic approaches.
BrightFocus Foundation	1-800-437-2423	brightfocus.org	Research funding and caregiver resources for Alzheimer's, macular degeneration, and glaucoma.
U.S. Department of Veterans Affairs (VA)	1-855-260-3274	caregiver.va.gov	Support services and programs for veterans with dementia and their caregivers.
Fisher Center for Alzheimer's Research Foundation		alzinfo.org	Alzheimer's research, caregiver education, and free resources.
Alzheimer's Association	1-800-272-3900	alz.org	Helpline, education, caregiver resources, local support networks.

www.ingramcontent.com/pod-product-compliance
Lightning Source LLC
Chambersburg PA
CBHW030517080526
44586CB00011B/233